# TIMOTHY HYMAN
## A YEAR WITH MAGGIE'S

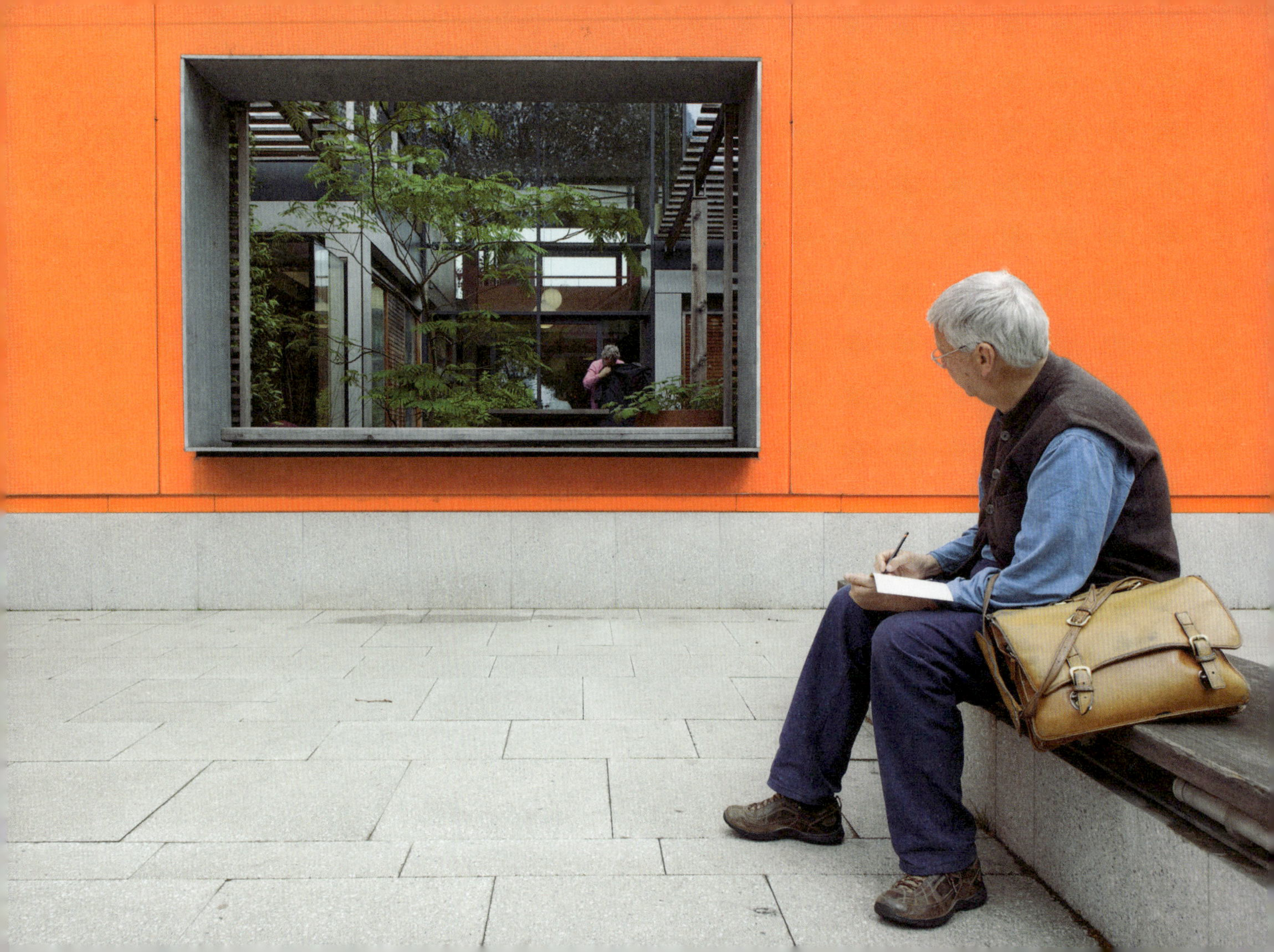

Timothy Hyman

# TIMOTHY HYMAN

## A YEAR WITH MAGGIE'S

For Ben
— thanks!
TH

Royal Academy of Arts *in association with* Maggie's

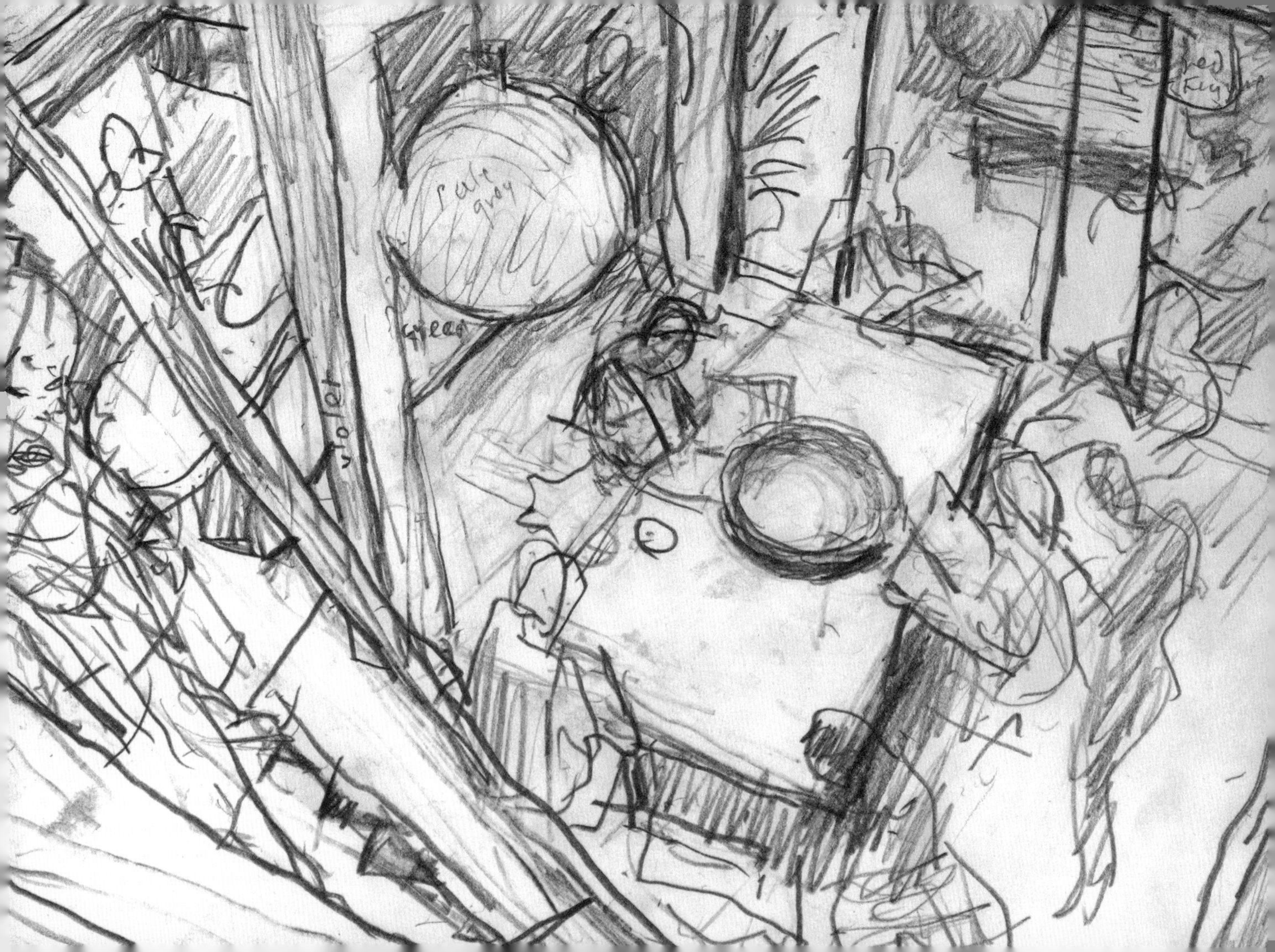
pale grey
green
violet
red

## FOREWORD

People come to Maggie's for help and support at a tough time in their lives. They have cancer or have had cancer (or love someone with cancer). However good their medical treatment, their world has been turned upside down. How will they live with this?

Without the capacity to hope, to imagine, to be creative, life with or without cancer is pretty meaningless. Maggie's aims to re-kindle people's belief in themselves, to help them imagine, create and hope again.

Tim's brief was to capture 'the life of the centre', and this is what he has done, quite wonderfully. His vigorous line, barely contained by the page, vividly describes the people and the places he draws… these people are amazing, full of life, full of character. Far from looking downbeat, they are engaged, energetic even. You can hear them talking, see them listening, watch their legs waving in the air in a yoga class.

I think Tim somehow thought he had missed out on the gritty bits. I don't agree with him. I can see gritty bits there too, but the people he has drawn are incredible. They are facing the worst that life can throw at them and rising to the challenge. This is what Maggie's is like, and what the people who come to Maggie's are like.

We are enormously grateful to Christopher Parish, Felicity Guinness and Stewart Heslop of the Cocheme Trust for seeing the potential of funding an artist's residency and, through this book, allowing us to share life at Maggie's with a wider audience.

Marcia Blakenham

## INTRODUCTION

*'To capture the life of the centre'*

The drawings at the core of this book came out of a painter's sixty visits to Maggie's cancer-caring centres. These informal havens allow those who are coming to terms with a cancer diagnosis to begin to access support and 'get back their lives'. The first Maggie's Centre opened in Edinburgh in 1996, using a blueprint for cancer caring laid down by Maggie Keswick Jencks during the eighteen months before her death from advanced breast cancer in June 1995. Since then the charity has commissioned a sequence of outstanding buildings, all modest in scale, sited alongside large NHS hospitals; many have been designed by major architects, often without fee.

In 2011–12 Timothy Hyman RA took up an artist's residency at the only Maggie's Centre then in London, located beside Charing Cross Hospital in the Fulham Palace Road. Designed by Richard Rogers in collaboration with Ivan Harbour, the building won the RIBA Stirling Prize for architecture in 2009. The extracts that follow from Timothy Hyman's first-person account are intended to provide a parallel narrative to his drawings, which have been selected from the much larger number he made during the year.

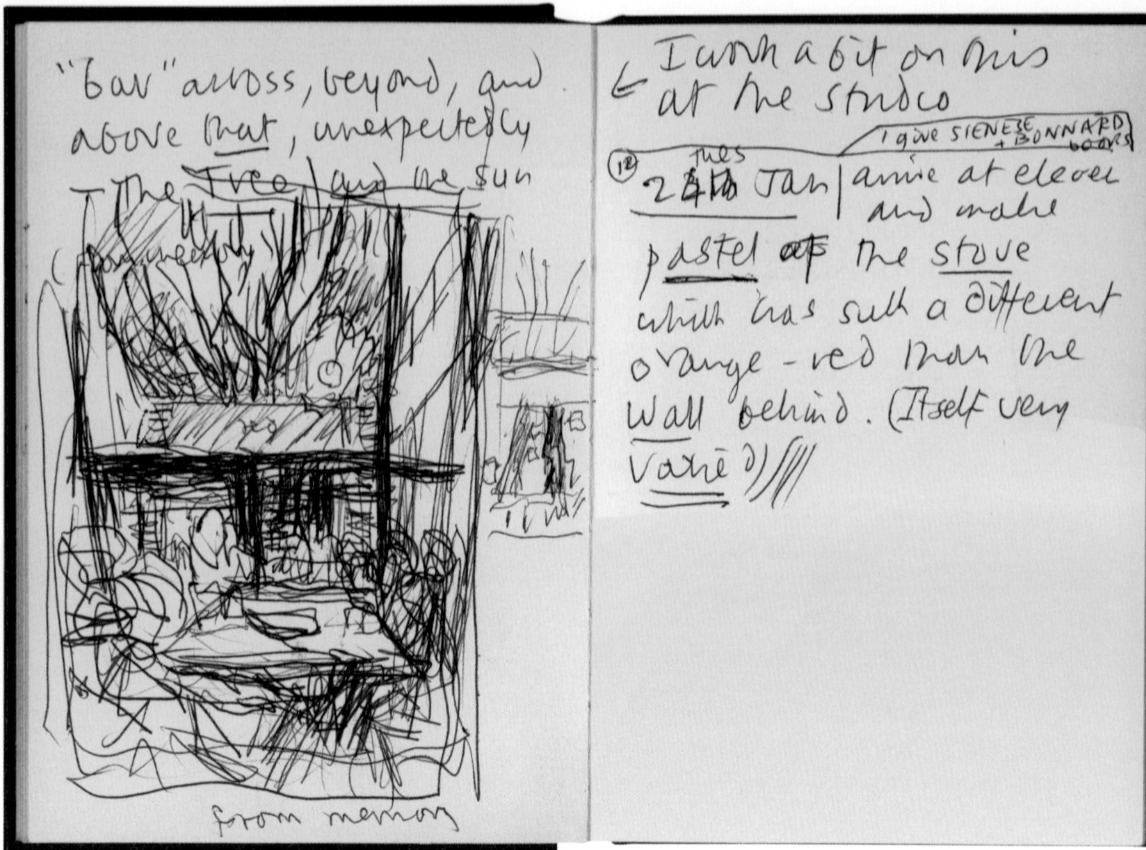
"bar" across, beyond, and
above that, unexpectedly
The Tree and the sun
from memory
← I work a bit on this
at the studio
I give SIENESE + BONNARD books
(12) Tues 24th Jan | arrive at eleven
and make
pastel of the stove
which has such a different
orange-red than the
wall behind. (Itself very
varied)

## SEPTEMBER 2011

A telephone call from Marcia Blakenham, a Board Member of Maggie's since the beginning: could I suggest a few artists who might be suitable for a residency now being set up at Maggie's cancer-caring centres? As the conversation deepens I grow enthusiastic: 'Whoever gets this role will find it a privilege!' And later, 'It sounds like the next best thing to being a war artist!' I come up with a few names, and say I will give it more thought. Then, just as I am about to ring off, Marcia says: 'Might *you* be interested?'

Over the following few weeks I find out more about the organisation: reading Maggie Keswick Jencks's own impassioned account, *A View from the Front Line*, composed just before her death in 1995; meeting Marcia at the Maggie's Centre; eventually, in November, going to the Maggie's offices, gorgeously set above the Thames, and signing the contract. Marcia already knows my drawings, and she sees this essentially as a drawing residency, equivalent to one day a week for a year. But it is Laura Lee, Maggie's Chief Executive (and formerly oncological nurse to Maggie herself), who clarifies the Maggie's ethos, and spontaneously comes up with my brief: 'To capture the life of the centre.'

## DECEMBER 2011

*Thursday 1 December*
My first session. I set out on a grey morning – though by the time I get to Baron's Court, the sun's out. As I walk through the familiar Margravine Cemetery, and then through the hospital, I remember my visits to Tony, my cancer-stricken twin brother, in 1999. Passing through the revolving doors into the chaotic entrance court I see the orange-red pavilion of Maggie's – a little Aesculapian temple – beckoning from a distance. It's 10 am and not many have arrived yet; I hover outside where the shadows of the trees are thrown by the low winter sun, dappling the orange wall in a marvellous way. I observe a young musician, large instrument strapped to his back, sitting on the bench, pensive, hesitating about whether to go in.... And then he straightens up and strides resolutely towards the entrance: later, just as I'm getting going upstairs, Marcia and then Laura too appear with the architect Steven Holl, who is about to design a new Maggie's Centre to be built at St Bartholomew's Hospital on the edge of the City. (We talk about the architect Louis Kahn and his paintings.)

Afterwards, sitting on a bench in the Margravine Cemetery, I say my prayers and tell myself: 'This is the kind of role I should have had at forty!'

But – mindfulness, mortality, now means so much more to me – I'm acquainted with grief, and with cancer – with the deaths of my twin, my parents, my friends.

But – you now draw more, and you often counterpoint architecture and figures; that's *why* they gave you the job.

But – Maggie's didn't exist when you were forty.

In any case – you weren't *ready* then.

*The Pensive Musician*

OVERLEAF *At the Entrance*

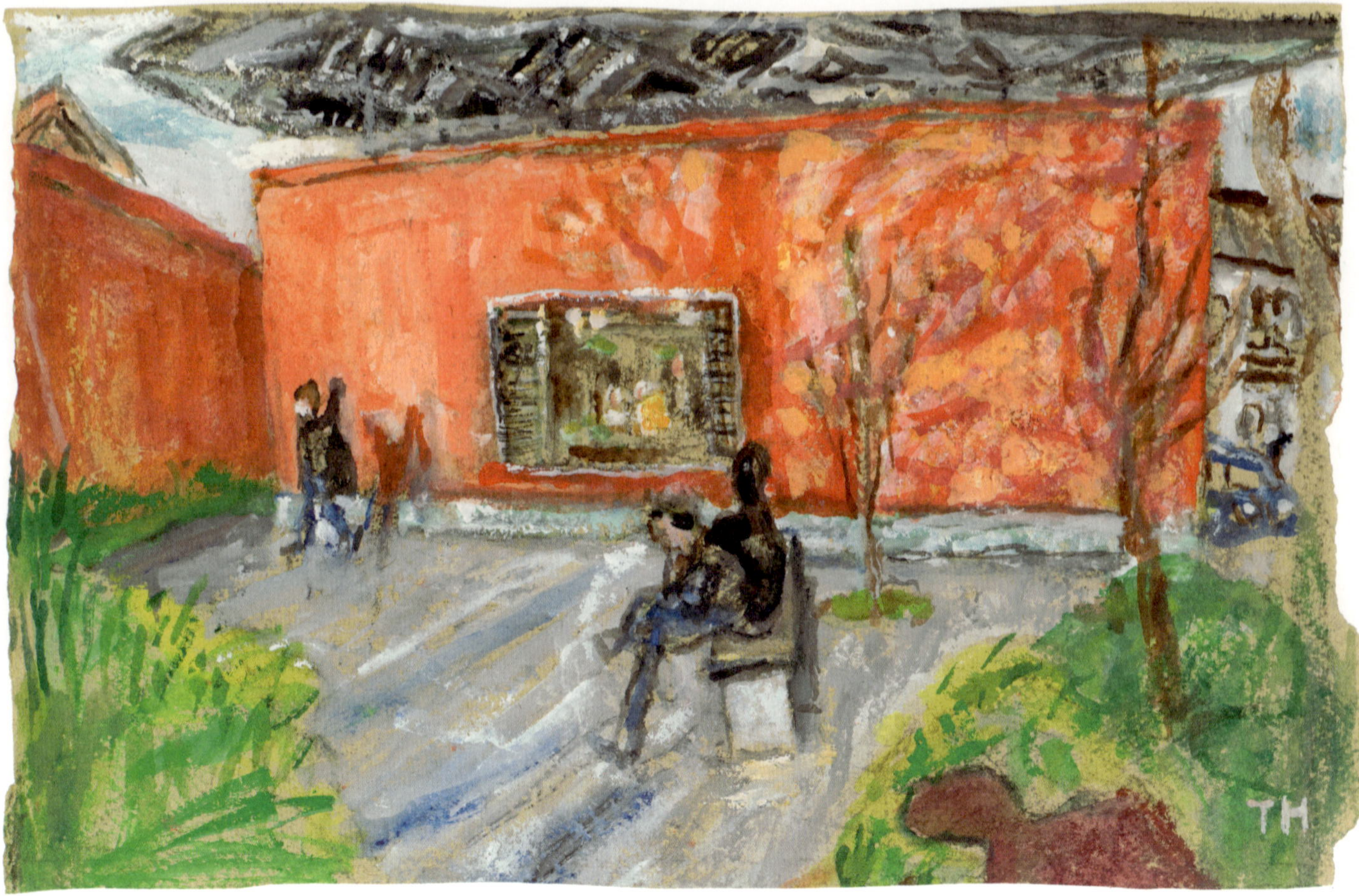
TH

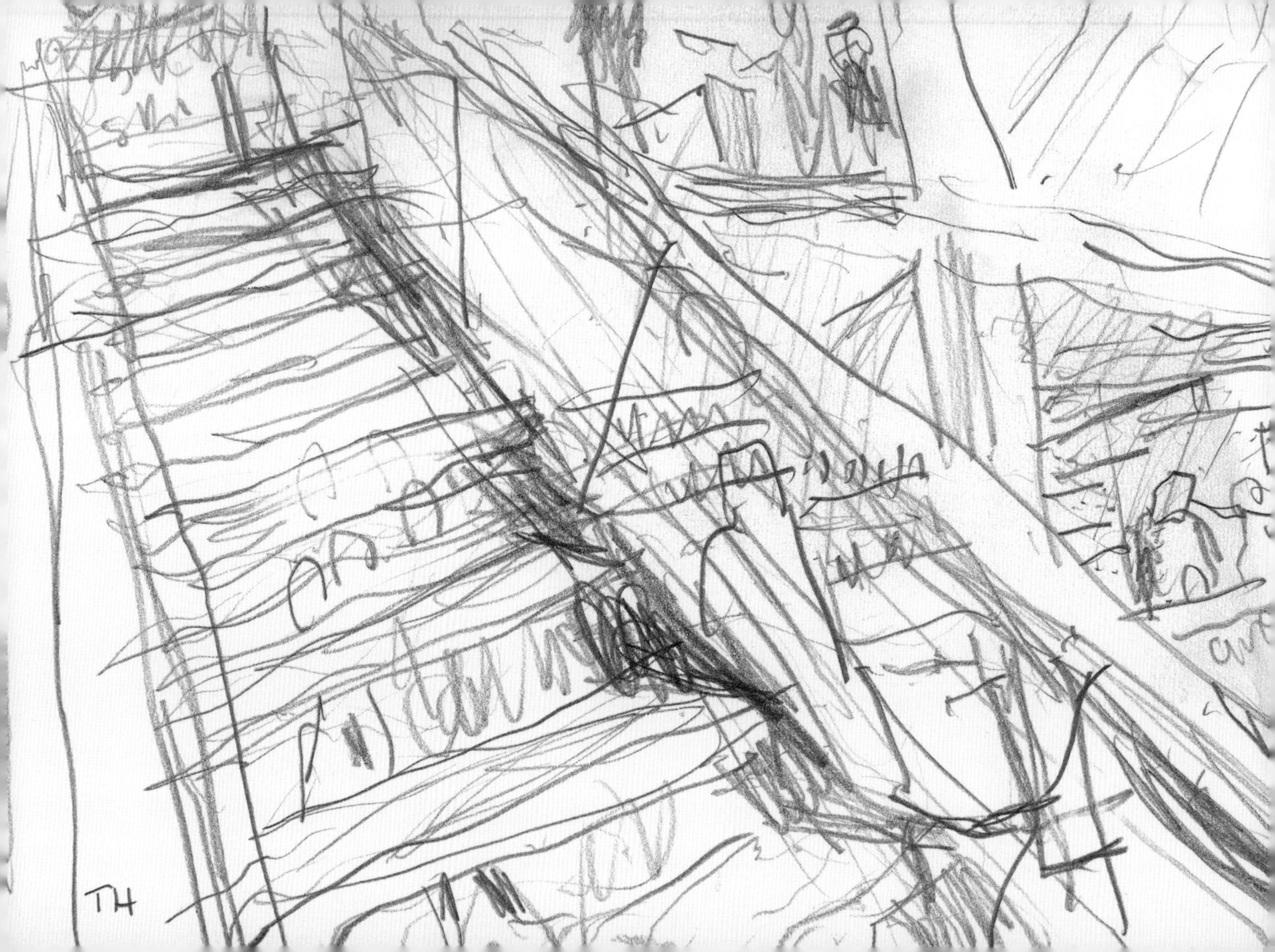
TH

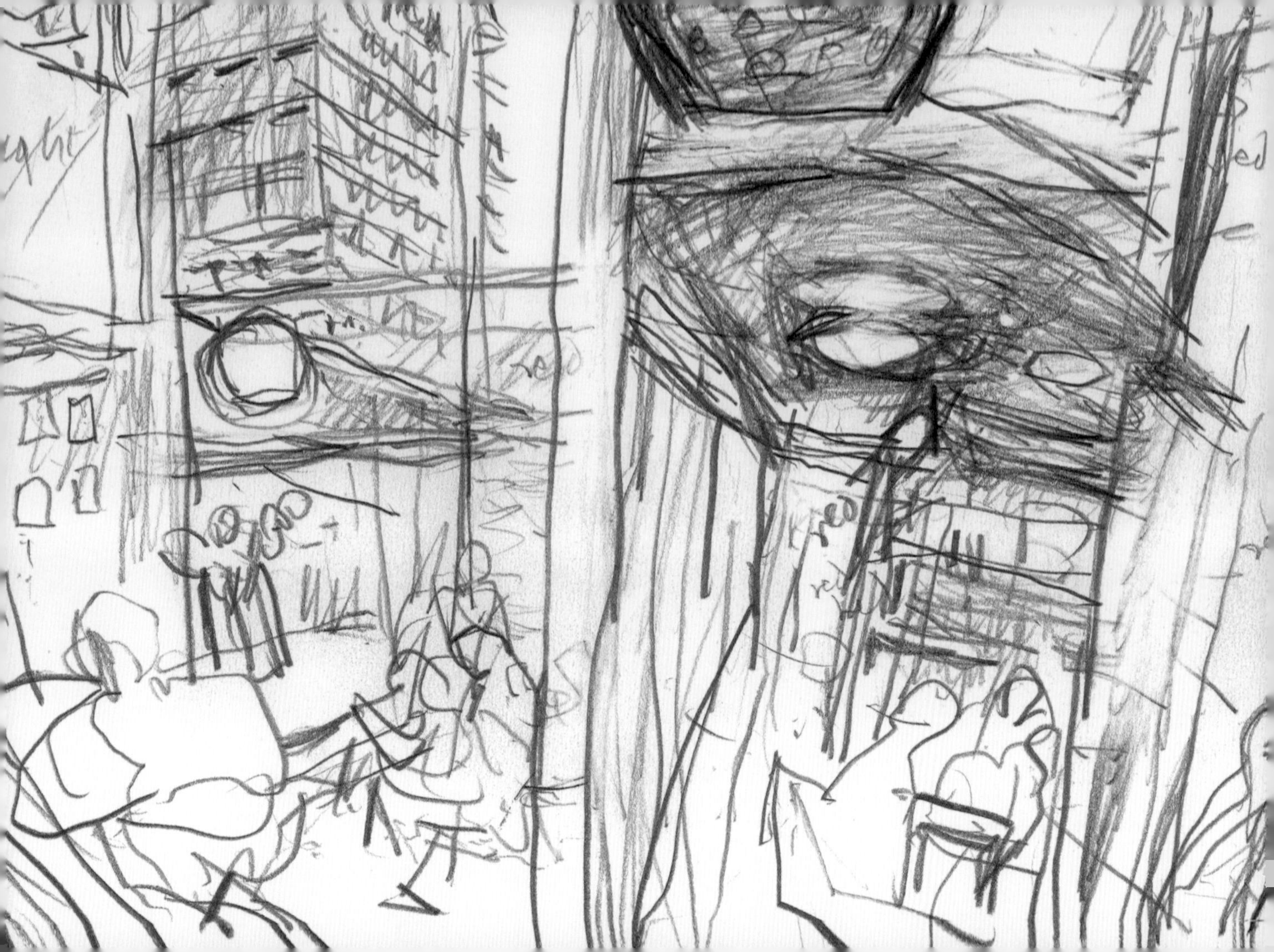
red
red

*Monday 5 December*

I've decided to log each visit in a small, separate notebook. I am introduced to the Prostate Group. They seem to accept my presence. A two-hour session follows with nutritionist Catherine (one woman to ten men). All of them are ALERT – a good class. They're not daunted but not in denial either. I *learn* a lot.

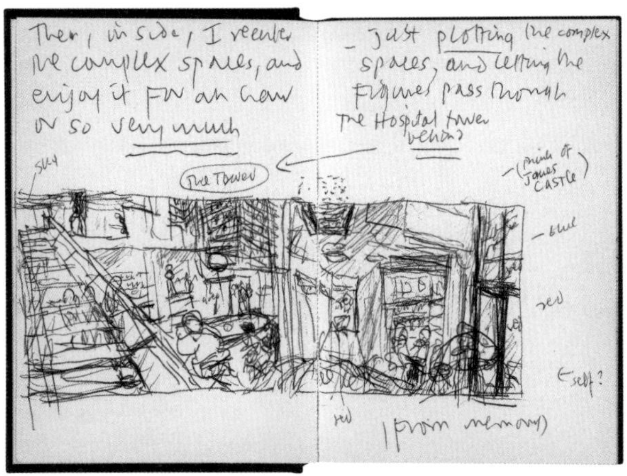


*At the Prostate Group I*

OVERLEAF *At the Prostate Group II*

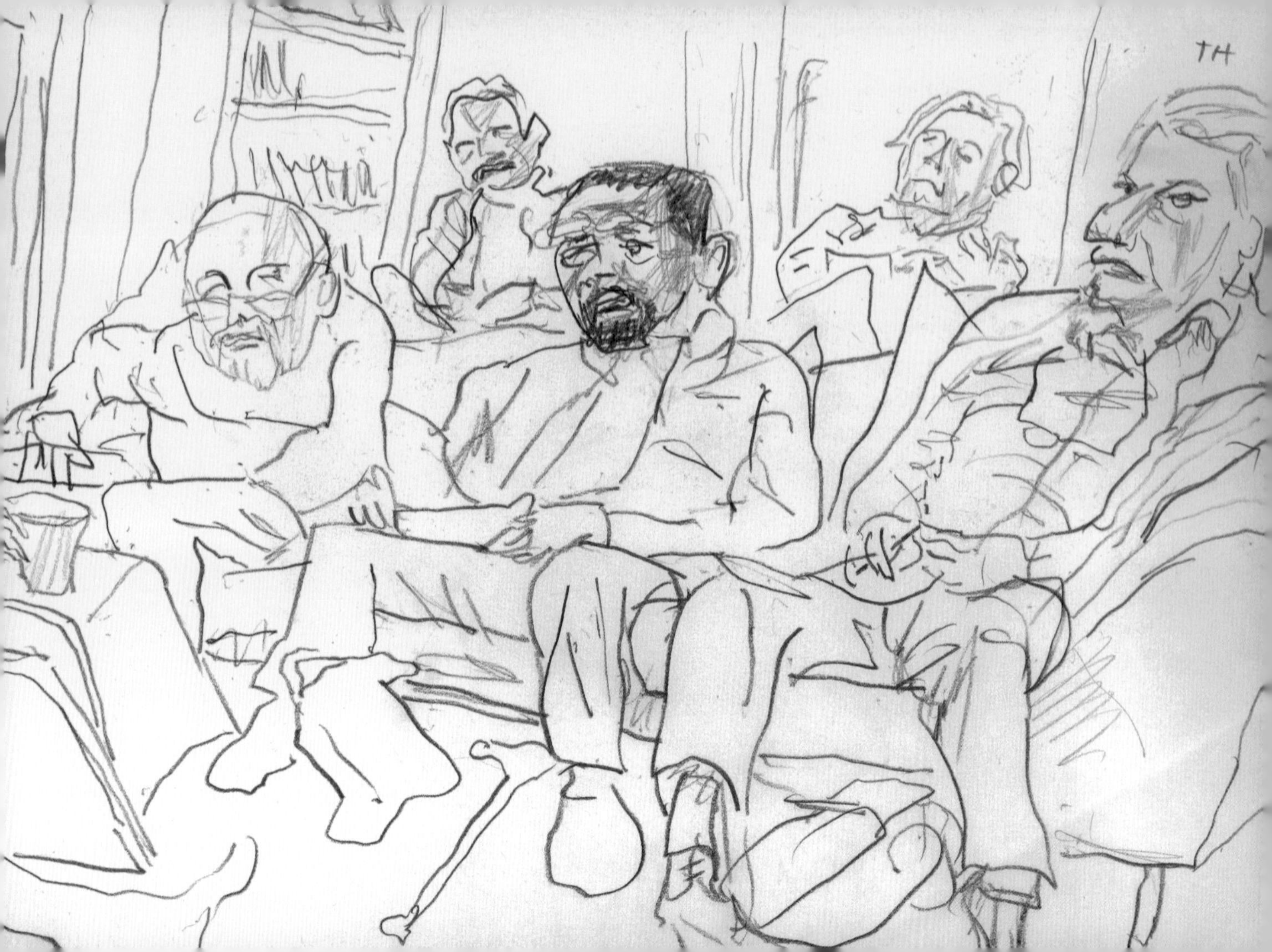
TH

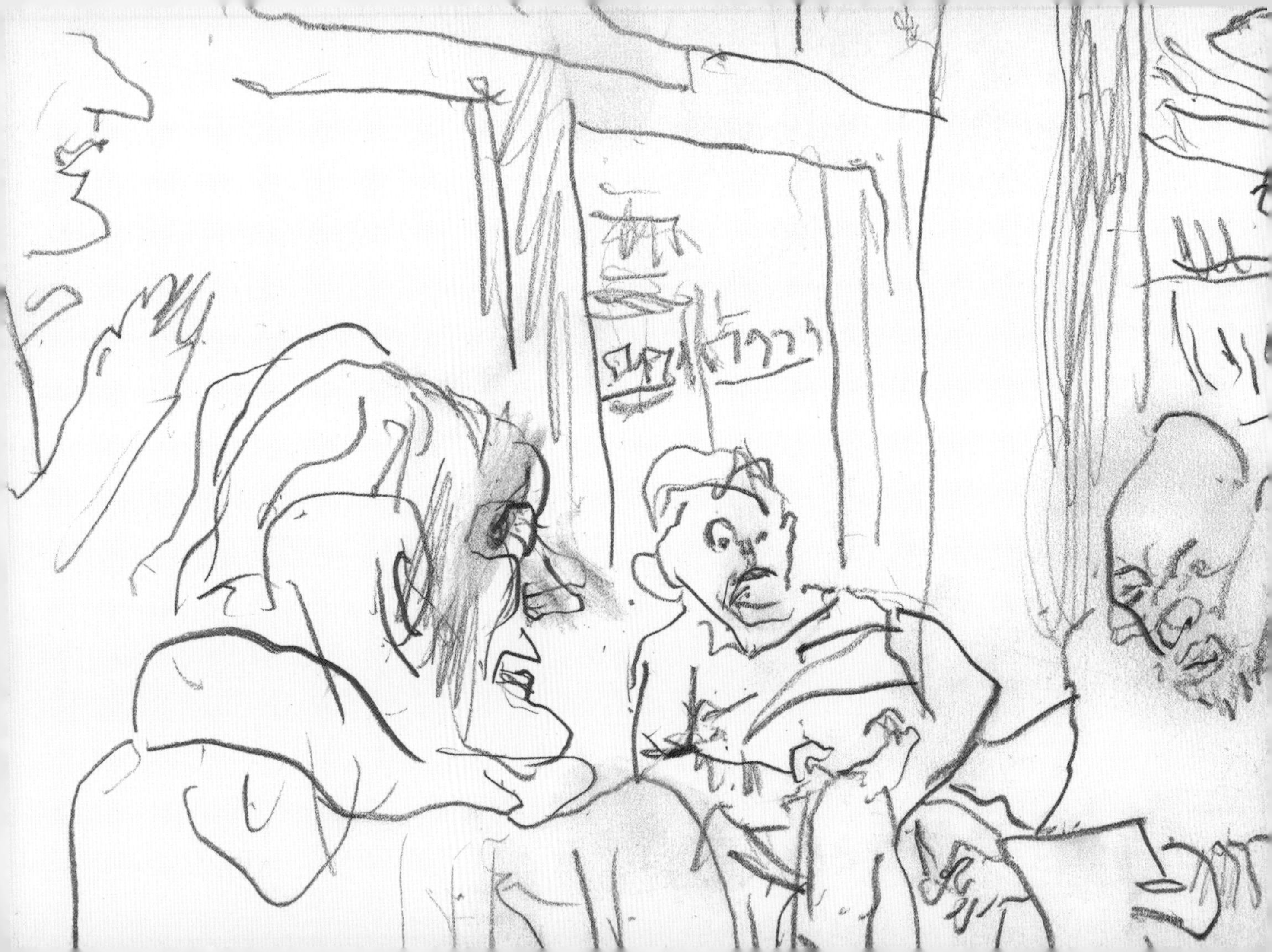

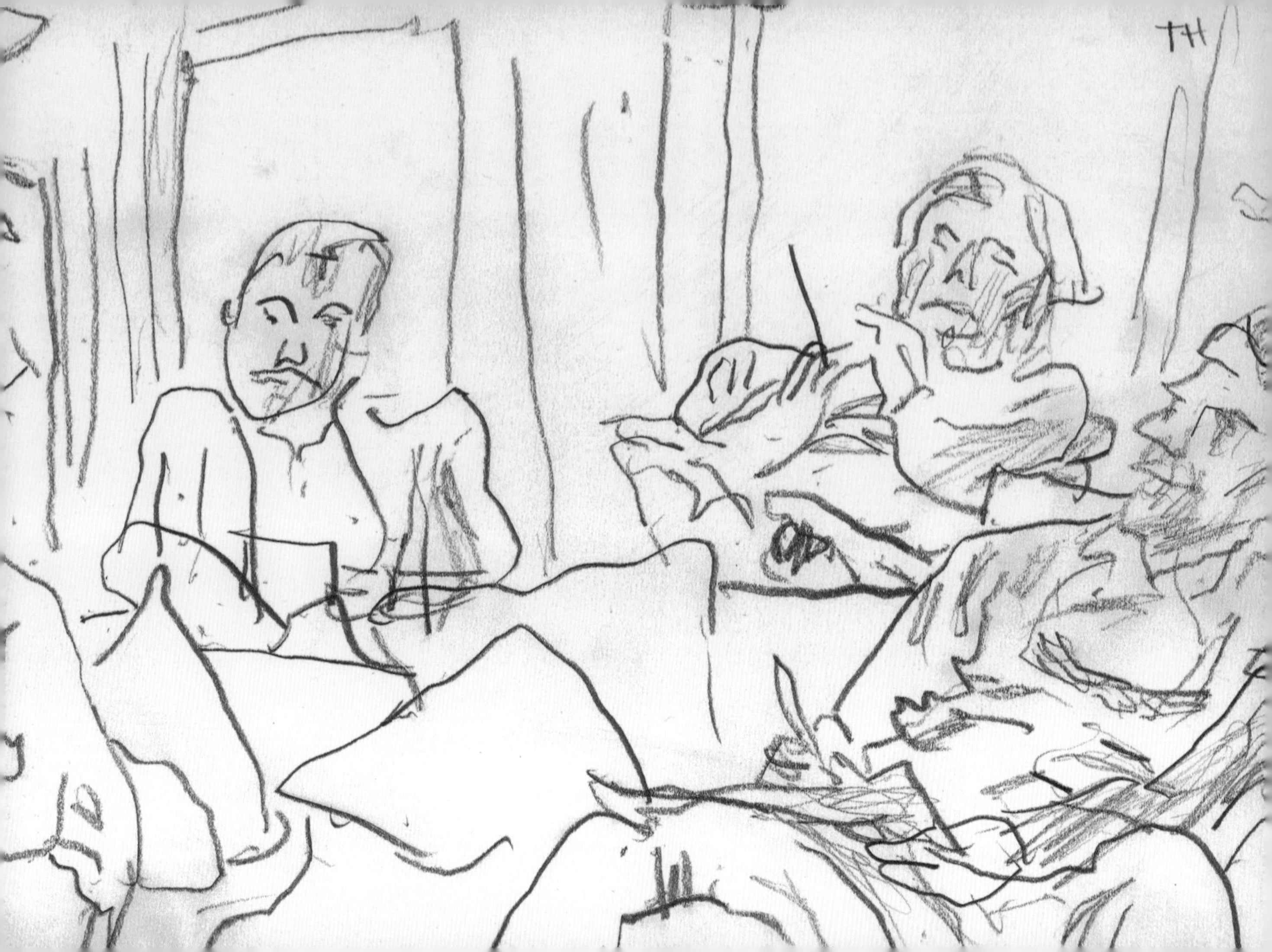
TH

*Wednesday 14 December*
I arrive in good time for the tai chi class, meeting the teacher, who comes from Hong Kong. He has a jutting, almost aggressive stance, and barks instructions: 'white crane', 'wings spread', 'cleaning windows'. I enjoy just keeping the pencil moving, and watching the class move too, each in a characteristic way: the talented Rasta guy with dreadlocks; the beautiful young Indian woman; the serious European, forty plus, in striped sweater and tunic; an Englishwoman who moves very well; and also an elderly Chinese, who keeps needing to rest. All are cancer 'victims'. And above them on the shelf a white ceramic BIRD watches us with its beady eye.

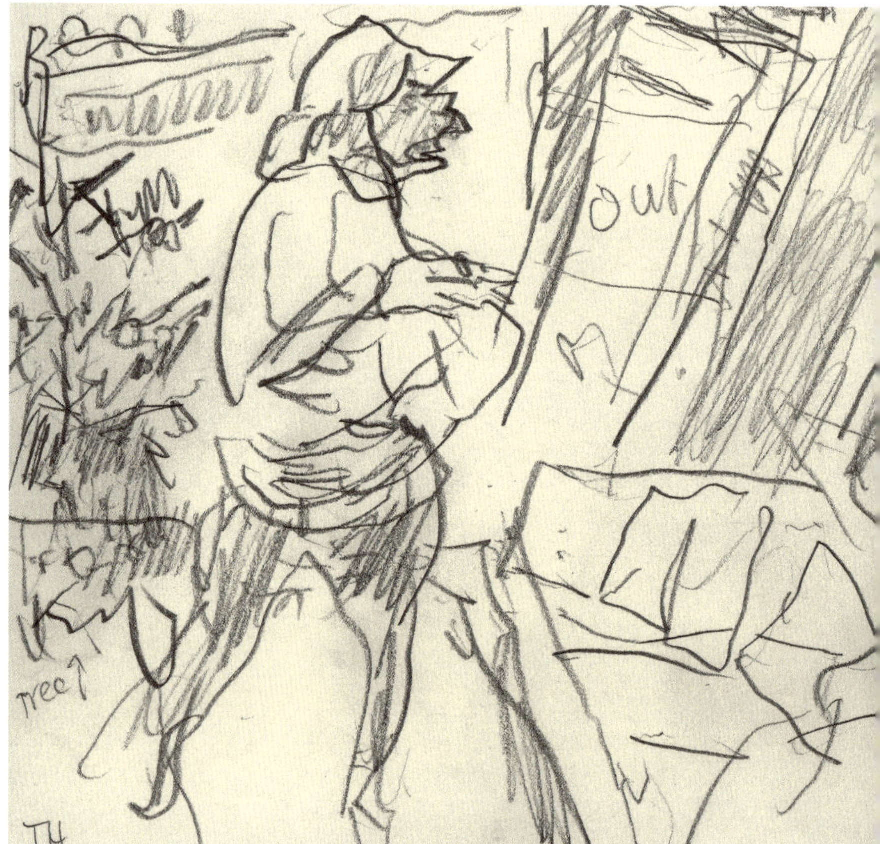

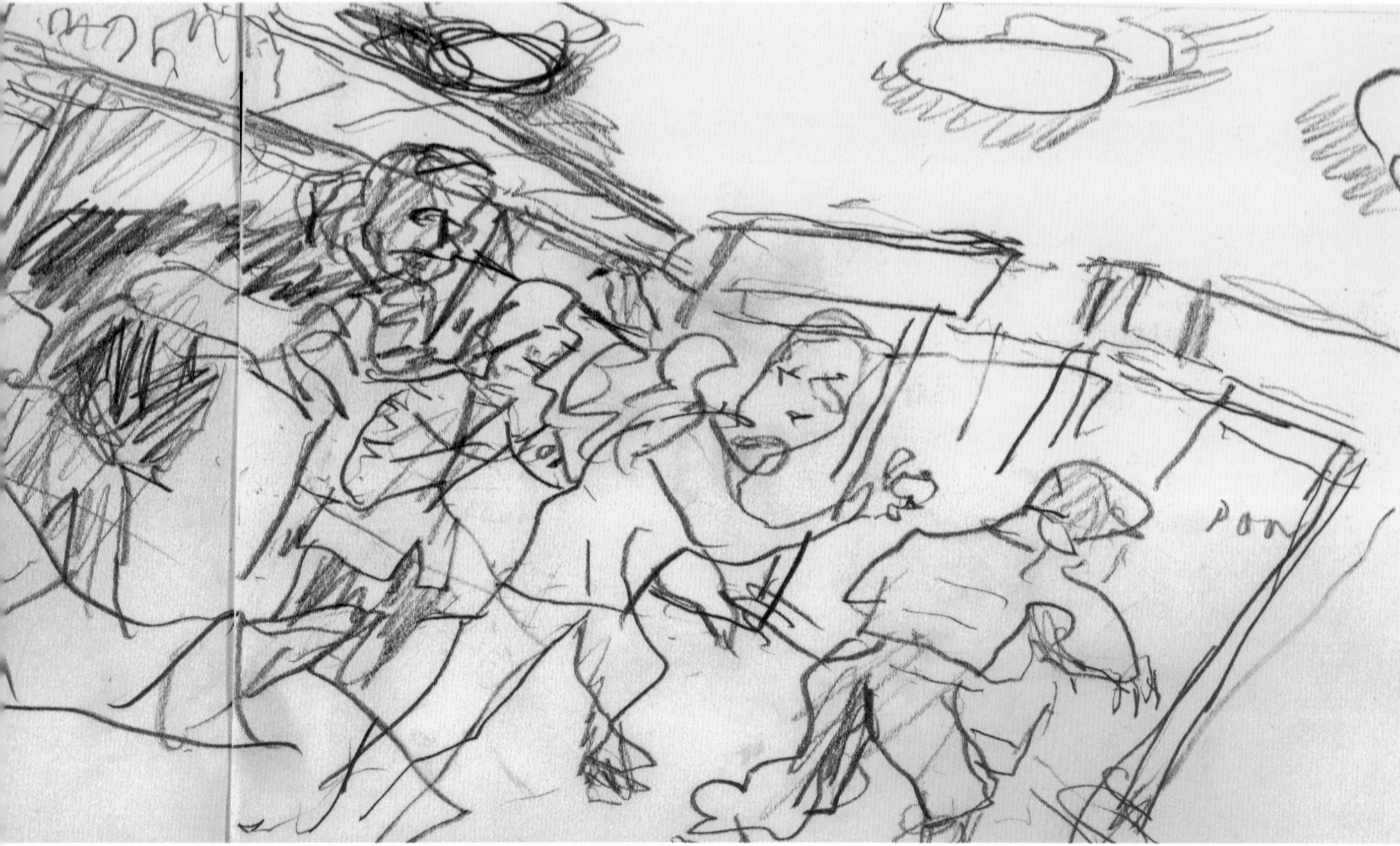


*Tai Chi*

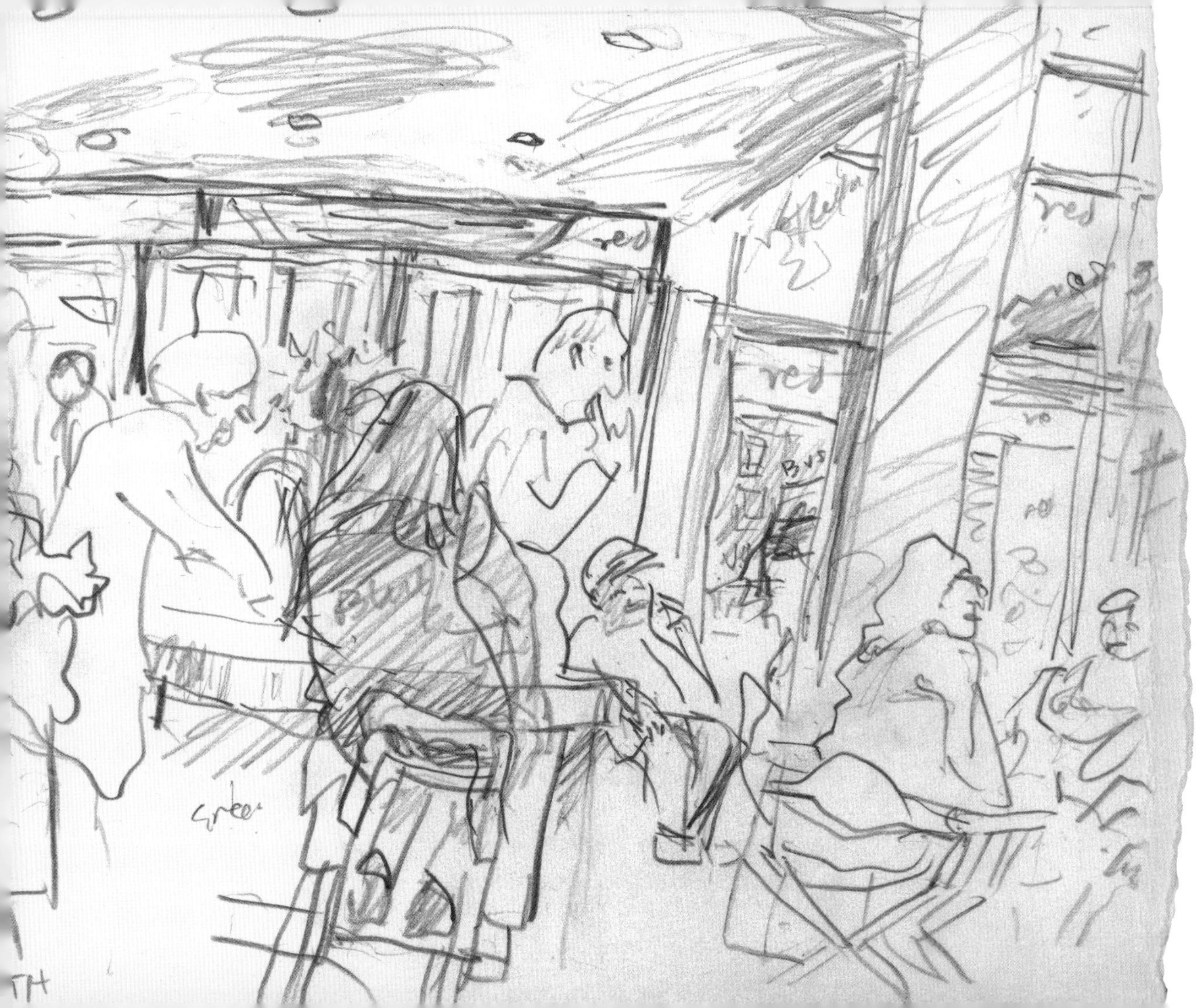
red
red
red
Bus
TH

*Monday 19 December*
After some good days' work in the studio, I set out to visit my twin brother Tony's grave in Brompton Cemetery on the twelfth anniversary of his death. Keyed up, emotional, at first I fail to find it, wandering with flowers in hand the whole vast length of the place in the rain. I am relieved to reach Maggie's and draw quietly, mindful of mortality.

*Wednesday 21 December*
I reach Maggie's before 10 am, and draw the group making Christmas wreaths at the big table upstairs. Then I draw the downstairs room looking down from on high. Later I attend the Christmas party, enjoying drawing and talking to several, including an interesting Indian woman named Rani, and a Dutchman, Nicholas, who studied at St Martin's.

*At the Christmas Party*

## JANUARY 2012

*Tuesday 11 January*
I am conscious of my shyness at the table – i.e. being there *without* drawing. I need to get in deeper – 'to confront the suffering'. I've sent an email listing my ideal dates and activities from the January programme, but Bernie Byrne, head of this Maggie's Centre, counters this: 'We need to sit down now and be more methodical, so you don't have wasted journeys.' I can understand her position: the danger that my presence might obstruct or shut down the very processes that these centres were built to facilitate, the struggle to accept but not be defeated by cancer. But, like a documentary filmmaker, I do need access, to *witness*; otherwise, I am the war artist 'embedded' in the regiment, but who is not permitted to draw those wounded in combat…

So far I have been enjoying the pleasurable plotting of intricate spaces, of how people dispose themselves across the sheet of paper, the notation of individual physiognomies.

The 'Invisible Man' – the fly-on-the-wall – hanging around, hanging out.

Most of the centre's users appear confident and well dressed.
Whatever the skeletons lurking, this *is* a positive place.

*At Maggie's: Winter Light*

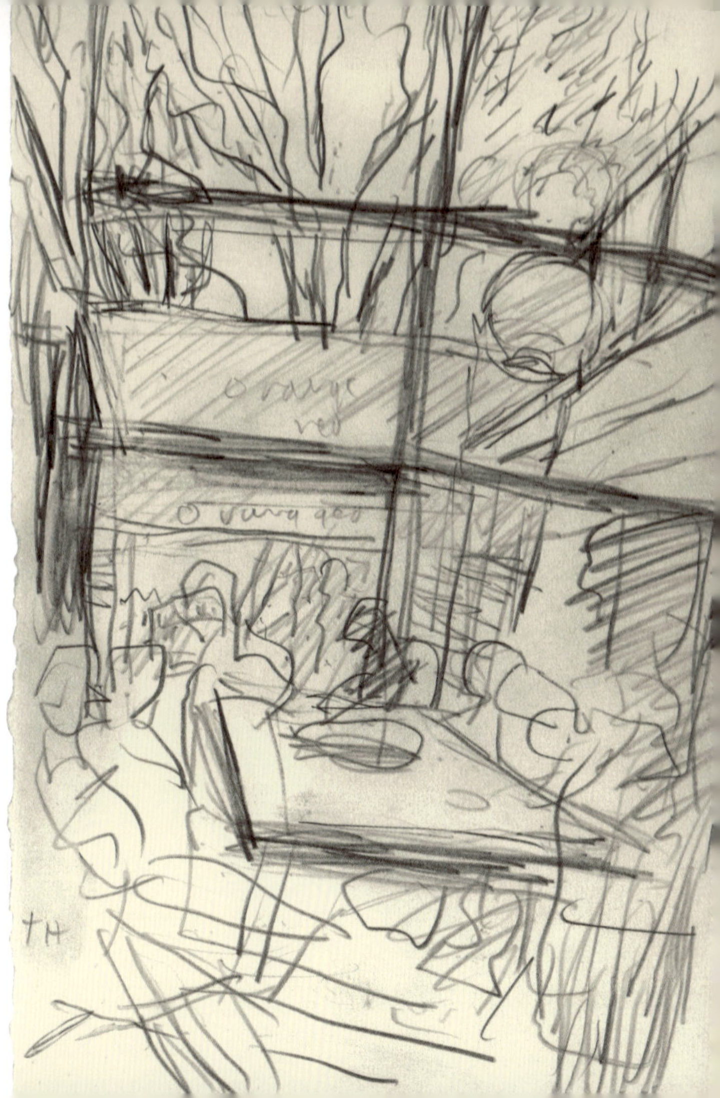

*Tuesday 17 January*
I arrive before 10 am, and attend the yoga class. This puts me at rather close quarters with an *entirely* female group. I sense some bristling at the male interloper. Later, I draw the table – the orange wall beyond, and above that, the tree and the pale winter sun.

*Tuesday 31 January*
Bernie sits me down with a team of four staff. Catherine, the psychologist, can't envisage being *natural* if I am present. But Robyn had noticed me drawing Mary kneeling beside a woman's chair; she thought this a 'classic' pose and was glad it was being recorded. It was legitimate for me to draw that transaction, *from a distance*.

Much that takes place at Maggie's does occur within the main space. But many interactions take place too within the confines of the consulting rooms – and I can see I can't expect to be witness to those. (And perhaps, after all, that isn't the point – it is the public space that is distinctive at Maggie's.)

At a relaxation session, I can *hear* the sound of my pencil; and when I attend the mindfulness class I don't draw. I've now met most of the staff here, as well as several part-time volunteers.

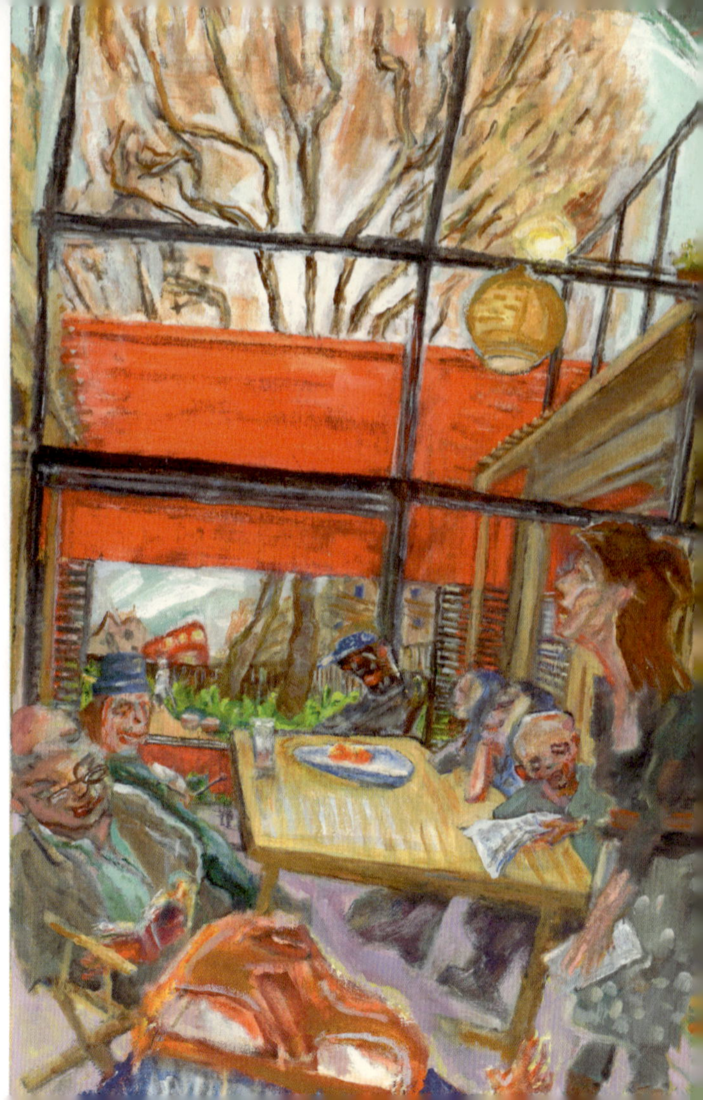

*At Maggie's: Winter Light*

OVERLEAF *A Little Aesculapian Temple*

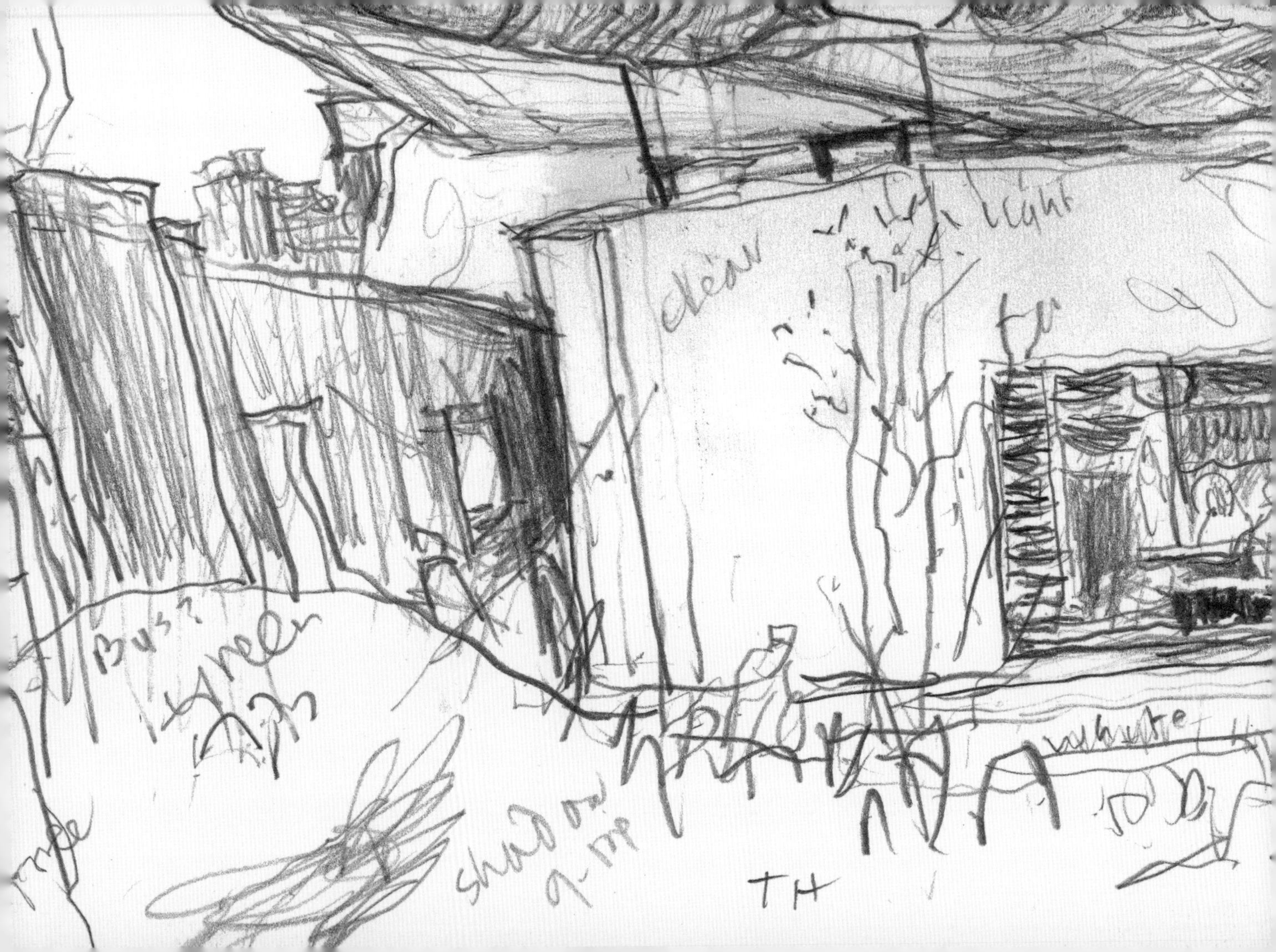
clear light
Bush
white
shadow
TH

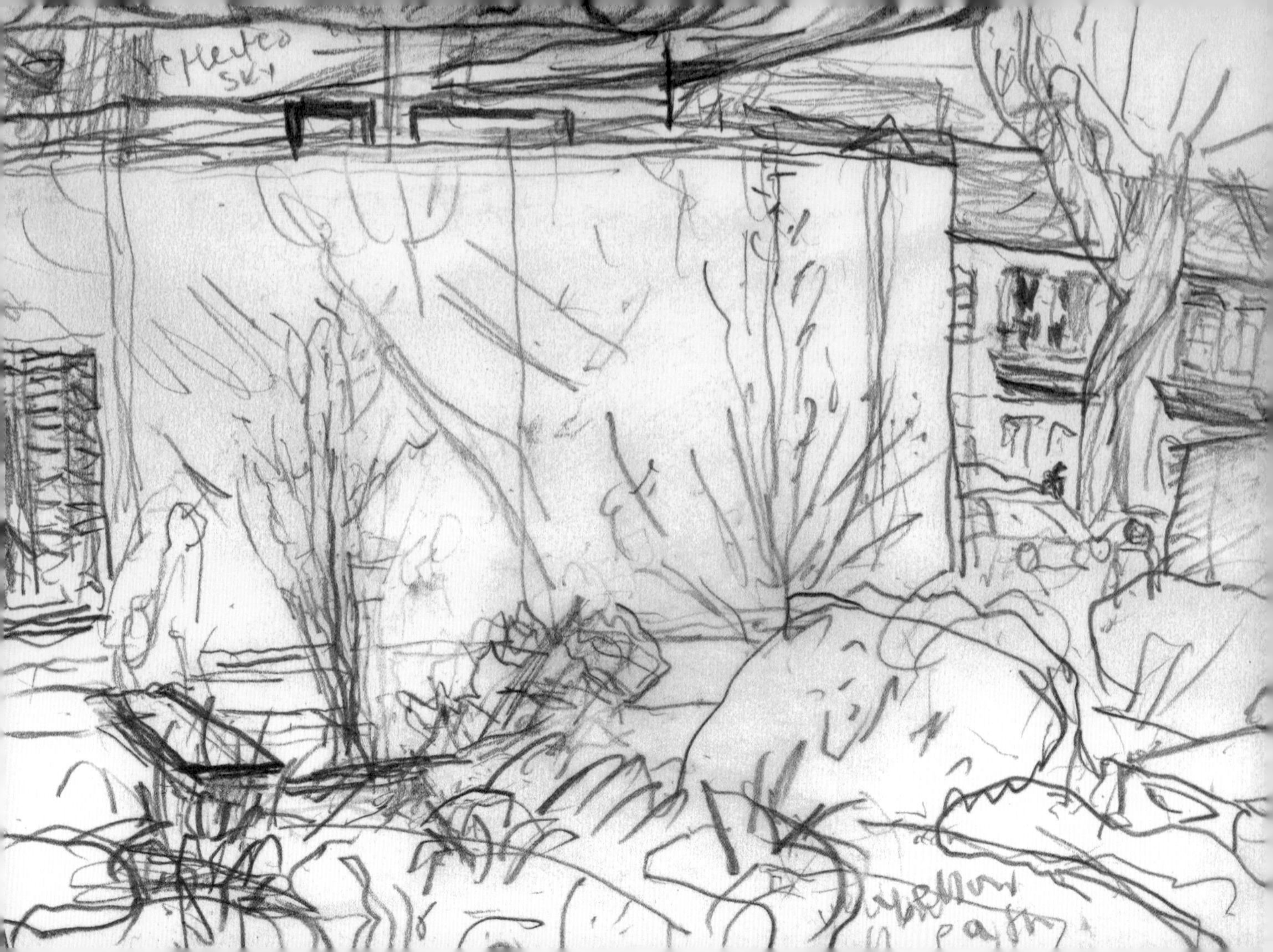
reflected
sky
yellow
path

## FEBRUARY 2012

*Thursday 2 February*
I arrive early, sit and draw at the table. Then, at about 11.45 am, I meet up with my wife Judith at the hospital, and escort her to the Maggie's Centre, seeing it through her eyes. A bright, sunny day on the sandy path – the brilliance of its winding, its planting, the illusion of Mediterranean or even tropical enchantment, rather like the transition in *The Wizard of Oz* from black and white to colour. We 'follow the Yellow Brick Road'. The receptivity of that orange-red to light is striking; we are both reminded of the Mexican architect Luis Barragán. At first this seems so small a building; what is unexpected is its *monumentality* as one steps into the entry passage, between the two orange walls, a temple precinct that creates significance, expectation.

*Monday 6 February*
I sit at the table (an Asian child is reading) as various men make their entrance for the Prostate Group. I rather admire them all, *bearing up*. The meeting turns out to be a discussion – they are filling in a questionnaire from a young Greek-Cypriot researcher, and this provokes some pretty frank exchanges. (A female nurse, hard-boiled, is present.) The underlying *sadness* surfaces. Despite Viagra, they lament the loss of *pleasure* (it lasts three hours, is priapic: 'You can do it, but it's *not the same*'). The other treatments sometimes lead to extreme fatigue

or incontinence. Some are very well informed. Many consultants apparently dismiss diet: '"It's too late," they say. "You might as well enjoy what's left."' Another voice: 'Yeah! "Start smoking!"' A drug showing signs of future success, promised to several of them, has just been rejected by N.I.C.E. They fret about the *uncertainty* of Chinese herbal treatments – when analysed, each packet's contents turn out to vary greatly. A Caribbean guy asks the nurse tentatively, 'Can you tell us about the new research into regeneration of the erectile muscles?' This is met with jeers from the far corner: 'You're dreaming, mate!', 'You're too old', 'It'll be fifty years before they get there.'

I just enjoy moving the pencil swiftly across them as they take notes; I'm accumulating these human beings as a 'collector-of-souls', in the phrase of the American portraitist Alice Neel, thinking of Gogol.

OVERLEAF *The Prostate Group III*

PAGES 32–33 *The Prostate Group IV*

TH

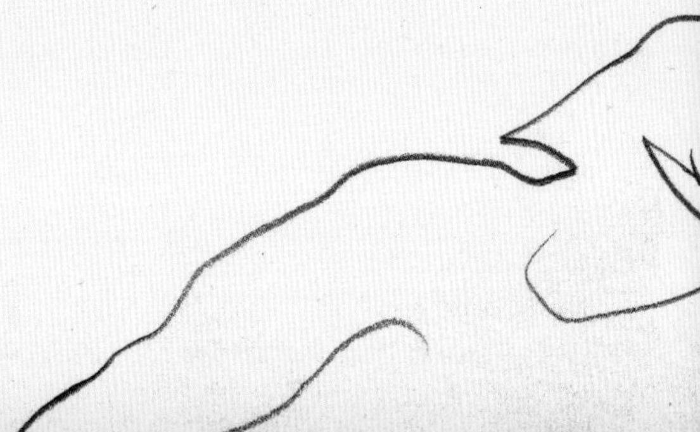

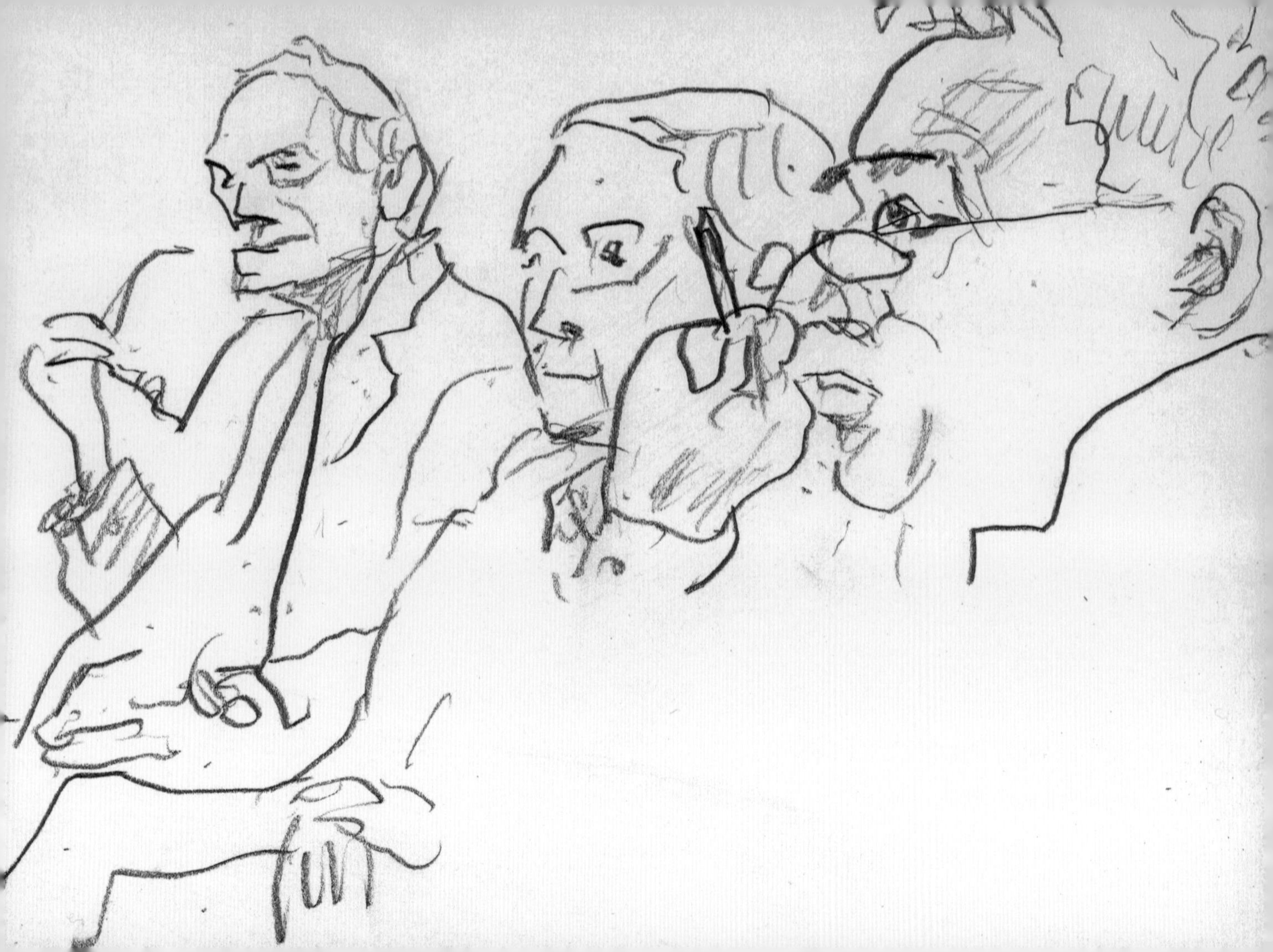

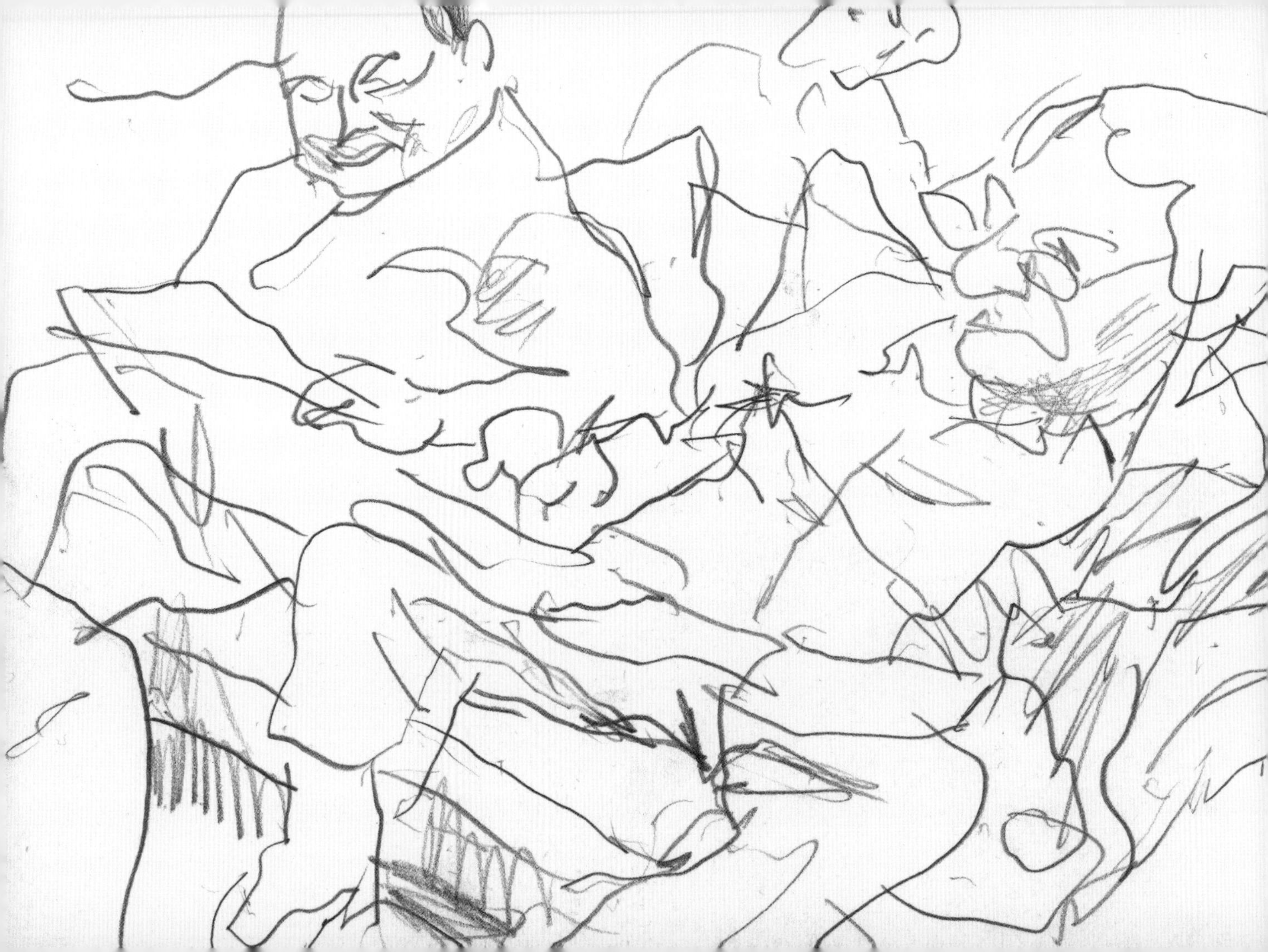

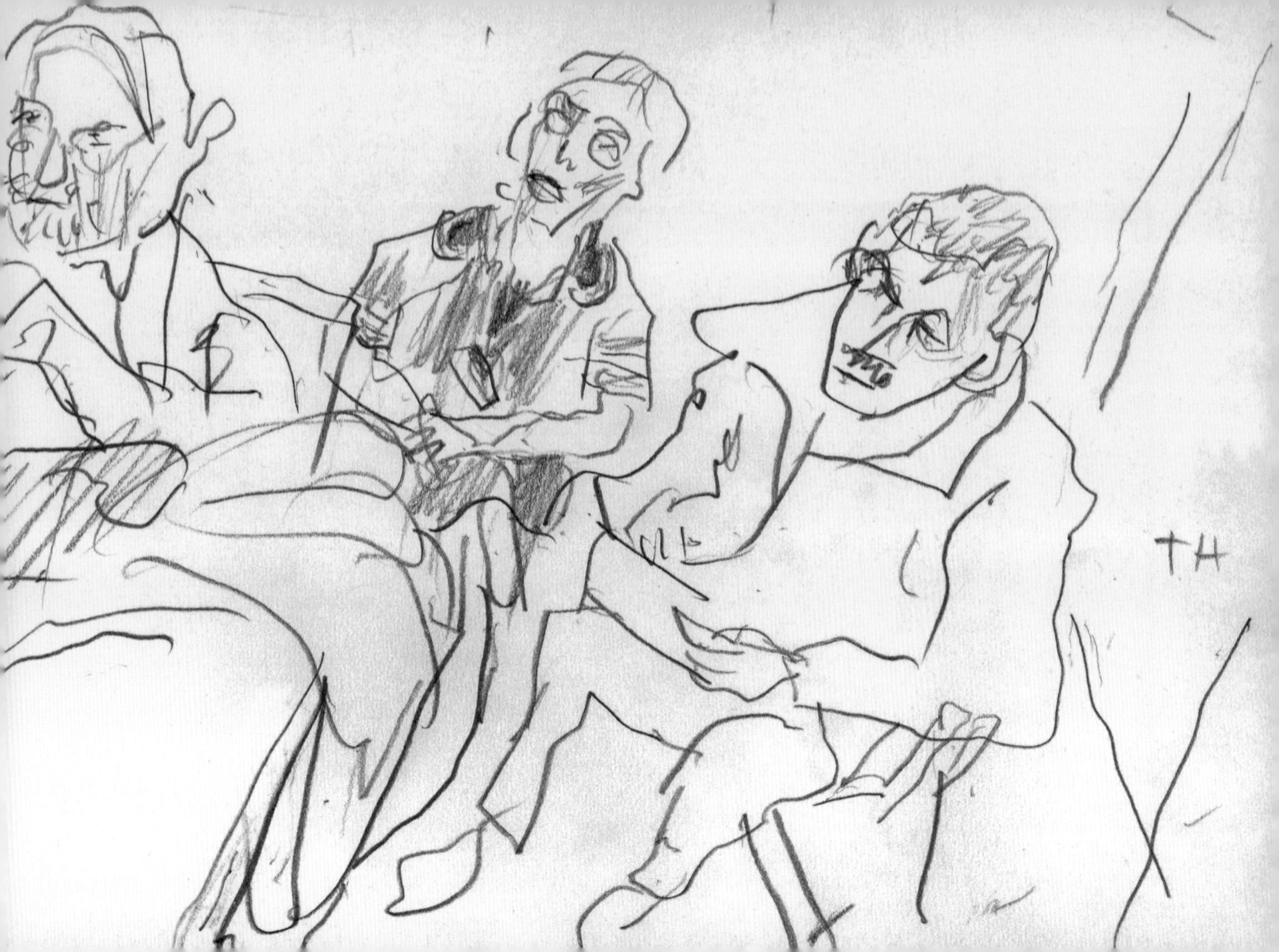
TH

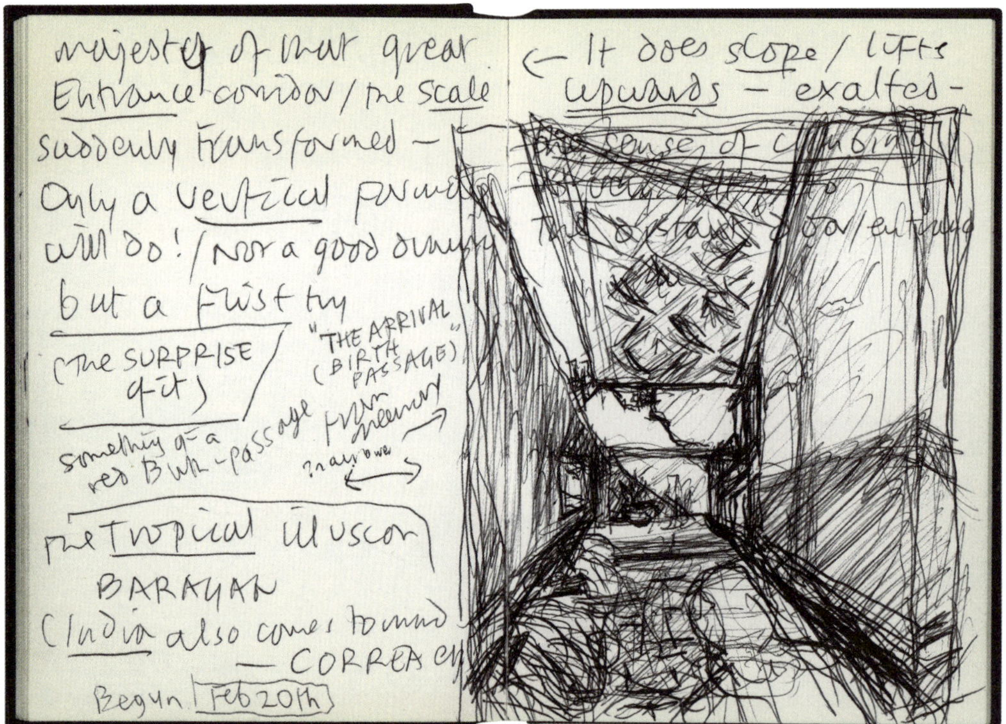
majesty of that great
Entrance corridor / the Scale
suddenly transformed –
Only a vertical format
will do! / not a good drawing
but a first try
(THE SURPRISE of it)
"THE ARRIVAL" (BIRTH PASSAGE)
from memory
something of a red Birth-passage
? narrower
the Tropical illusion
BARAYAN
(India also comes to mind
– CORREA
Begun Feb 20th
← It does slope / lifts
upwards – exalted –

*Thursday 16 February*
I arrive just before 11 am – and, immediately, on the yellow path, SEE it all anew – an epiphany – beginning with the view (of people around a table) through the deep 'hole' in the orange wall. The resulting drawing is among the most fully realised so far. I try to get the sense of Nature all around – and the spring of the roof – and a little glimpse of the everyday world beyond.

Then, almost immediately after, I also feel and see the majesty of that great entrance corridor, its scale suddenly transformed. For this, only a vertical format will do! (Richard Rogers wrote of 'a place that lifted the soul': the paved path does actually slope upwards, giving one a feeling of exaltation, the sense of *climbing* step by step towards the distant entrance.)

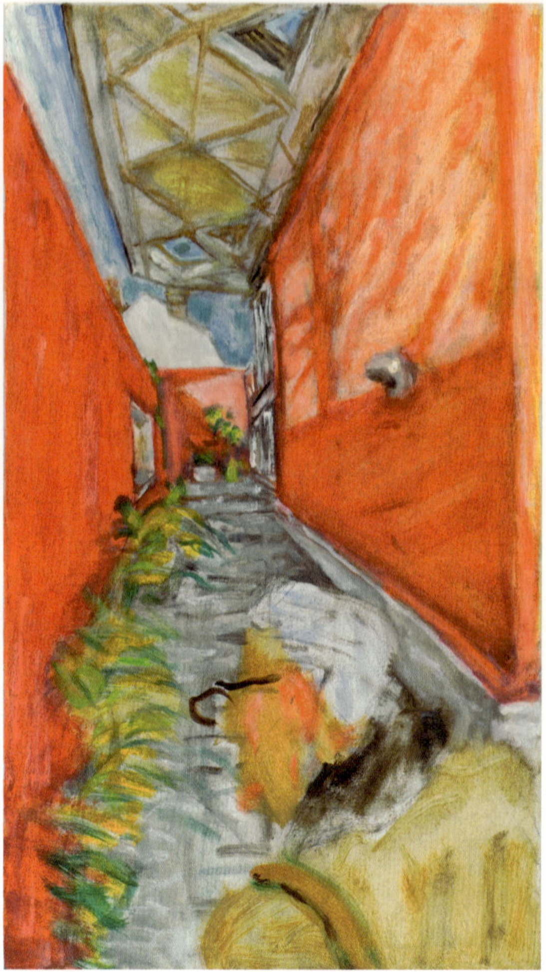

*The Arrival*

*Tuesday 21 February*

Over Sunday and Monday I've begun a small oil, *The Arrival* (p. 35); and also, in watercolour and gouache, a memory of the musician I saw on my first visit (p. 11), whom I privately call 'Tamino', after the desperate young man from *The Magic Flute*, hesitating outside the Masonic Temple.

I sit at the table, demurely, beside one of several imposing, matronly ladies. When I get up to make a hot drink, she too leaps up; she turns out to be E, ex-wife of P. I knew and rather admired her thirty years ago, when she was a fierce, proud feminist, challenging male assumptions, giving as good as she got. She's had three surgical interventions and endless chemo- and radiotherapy sessions – a year of her life lost. With help from Maggie's, E is trying to pull herself together. She attends yoga and relaxation classes here. I suggest the therapeutic act of DRAWING – and we have an informal mutual drawing session in the empty back room, chatting all the time. Hers is better than mine.

*Wednesday 29 February*

After yesterday's teaching at the Slade, I feel a bit drained, but sit straight down at the table *without drawing* – i.e. trying to be open, to engage. Four women are talking, two of them black, but I fail to enter their conversation. When the tai chi class comes out, I'm still sitting quite companionably – a cake has been baked, and I'm given a piece – when I recognise Rani, the bright Indian woman who chatted with me at the Christmas party. She's complimenting another woman on her

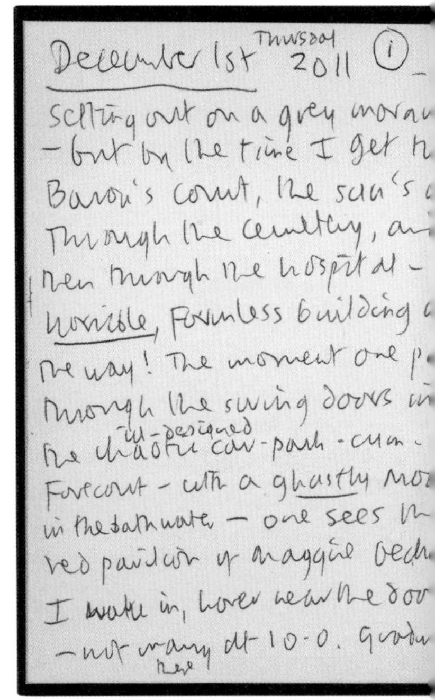

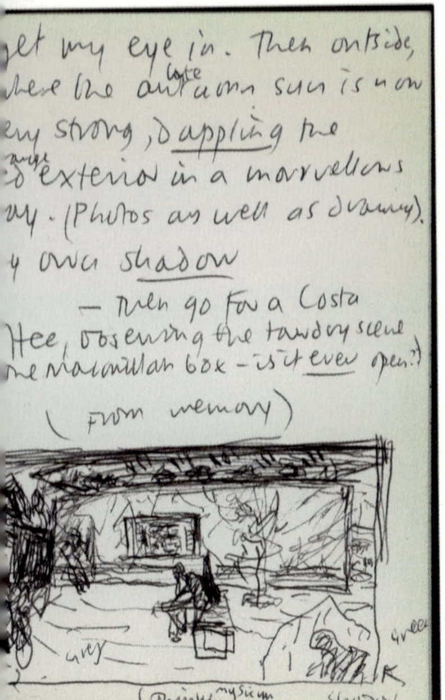


progress, generally exuding positiveness, and I ask her how she is getting along. But her response is not the conventional one: she embarks on an amazing hour-long account of all that has gone wrong in the two months since last we talked. A new tumour, a side-effect of her drug treatment; and after three years of close and friendly contact with her surgeon as one of his 'successes', he no longer replies to her emails. She expresses her fear and distress. At first she's standing, but when she gets further on into her narrative, she sits. 'I love my life … I don't want to be a footnote in *The Lancet*.' I listen, not putting my oar in too much.

## MARCH 2012

*Friday 6 March*

It turns out my elder brother Nicky now has lymphoma. I am currently re-reading Thomas Mann's *The Magic Mountain* after forty years – and suddenly seeing the parallels. I'm 'just visiting' the cancer ward (as Hans Castorp was the tubercular) only to discover that the enemy is much closer to home than I'd thought. (I've offered to 'introduce' Nicky at Maggie's, but he's already found help elsewhere.) Today, I'm trying to take stock of my work here so far – photocopying drawings for the Cocheme Trust, who have funded my residency – and to see for myself. I make appointments and commitments, but there is a slight loss of momentum, although I do run into E again, and we have another drawing session.

*Tuesday 20 March*
I am back, renewed, from a week with Judith in Naples. Along the path, everything is now blossoming, foliage has shot up and the door is open to the courtyard; a spring transformation. I have an appointment with Y – we start outside, but it is still a little too cold. At first she just *poses* – but I persuade her to begin drawing and immediately she really gets into it, and does an excellent drawing of me. We spend two sustained hours drawing together. I try to get something of her hex-appeal – spooky, doomy, but also quite *funny*. I like her.

Later, I photograph the semi-opaque window opposite the entrance, which now has odd, beautiful shadows, of foliage as well as the dimly seen figures and cars in the street – a reminder of the other world out there. It's one of the most poetic 'moments' of this building, but I'm not sure I can do anything with it.

*Wednesday 28 March*
An interesting visit; I arrive about 1 pm and sit down at the table. It's a bright day, the door is open and it's warm. I let the conversations flow around me. A nice Caribbean woman, here on her mother's behalf, offers a falafel to a pallid male stranger; he immediately opens up about prostate – the incontinence, the impotence. Amazing. Then a very bubbly woman at the table chats with the psychologist; the upbeat mask fades – and she comes right out with the horror: 'All my dignity – lost – and I'll never get it back…' Meanwhile I've started drawing in pastel. I don't think I did *art* today, but I did focus…

## APRIL 2012

*Monday 2 April*

I arrive before noon for the monthly Prostate Group, and it turns out they don't have a 'speaker', though about fourteen have turned up. Nigel is somewhat taking charge. A new visitor arrives in a wheelchair – in a bad way, but clearly helped by the camaraderie, the frankness of these exchanges. *All* have at some point been at death's door with 'aggressive' prostate cancer, and some have had it for twelve years. The most unselfconscious describes to me the moment of diagnosis, his clinical isolation. (He'd refused his daughter's offer to come over as he just wanted to sit alone.) And then the defiant reflex: 'I'll go out and have a fag and a couple of drinks.' In practice, most of the men who attend this group are in remission; there is much talk of PSA counts, with huge disparities. Yet they have 'entered the land of illness', and much of their energy is now spent investigating their options – the different gurus and practitioners and their clinics. We hear of Mark Emberton, who is signing people up for a new drug treatment, and will visit next Thursday. (I will aim to be there.) It turns out that only two of the group have been contacted about this. On what grounds have they been 'selected'? Elaine, our very capable convenor, tries to calm the situation. All experience nausea, incontinence, vomiting and exhaustion, but they do emerge from it – and, on this evidence, deepened and 'better' human beings. Even after surgery, the latent cancer may spread to the bones or other parts of the body. Risks are associated with these new treatments, according to one elderly military man. His son says: 'Don't do it, Dad, it could mess you up, it's too uncertain.' Another says blurrily, 'It gives you another two or three months' – i.e. of life. Nigel says: 'We lost three last year.' They all do feel the need for advice. Yet the spirit of this group is unbroken, resolutely hopeful, amusing. Alive!

*Thursday 12 April*

The Prostate Group are being briefed about a possible new course of treatment by Professor Mark Emberton. I get permission to draw. He speaks very well about medical ethics, opening with the statement 'All treatment is harmful'. ('We have to prove effectiveness, in order to justify any treatment – which may well cause damage, and may carry risks.') He examines the ethical issues of 'random' or 'targeted' new treatments, and the scandal of non-publication, i.e. of 'failures', and of biased or unrepresentative human samples (e.g. only white middle-class patients – or young male prisoners). So many tests do fail because participants drop out, or choose not to continue – not just in the UK, but everywhere. There is a possibility of a prostate breakthrough, though perhaps not in the age group mostly represented here (including me). I warm to Emberton – he is a real communicator, frank, forthright and unpompous. These new research projects would be thwarted in America by the money issue – in private medicine, a specialist loses income if a patient leaves in order to participate in a research project. By implication, the current Tory privatisation of the NHS could impede future research.

*Mark Emberton Talks to the Prostate Group I*

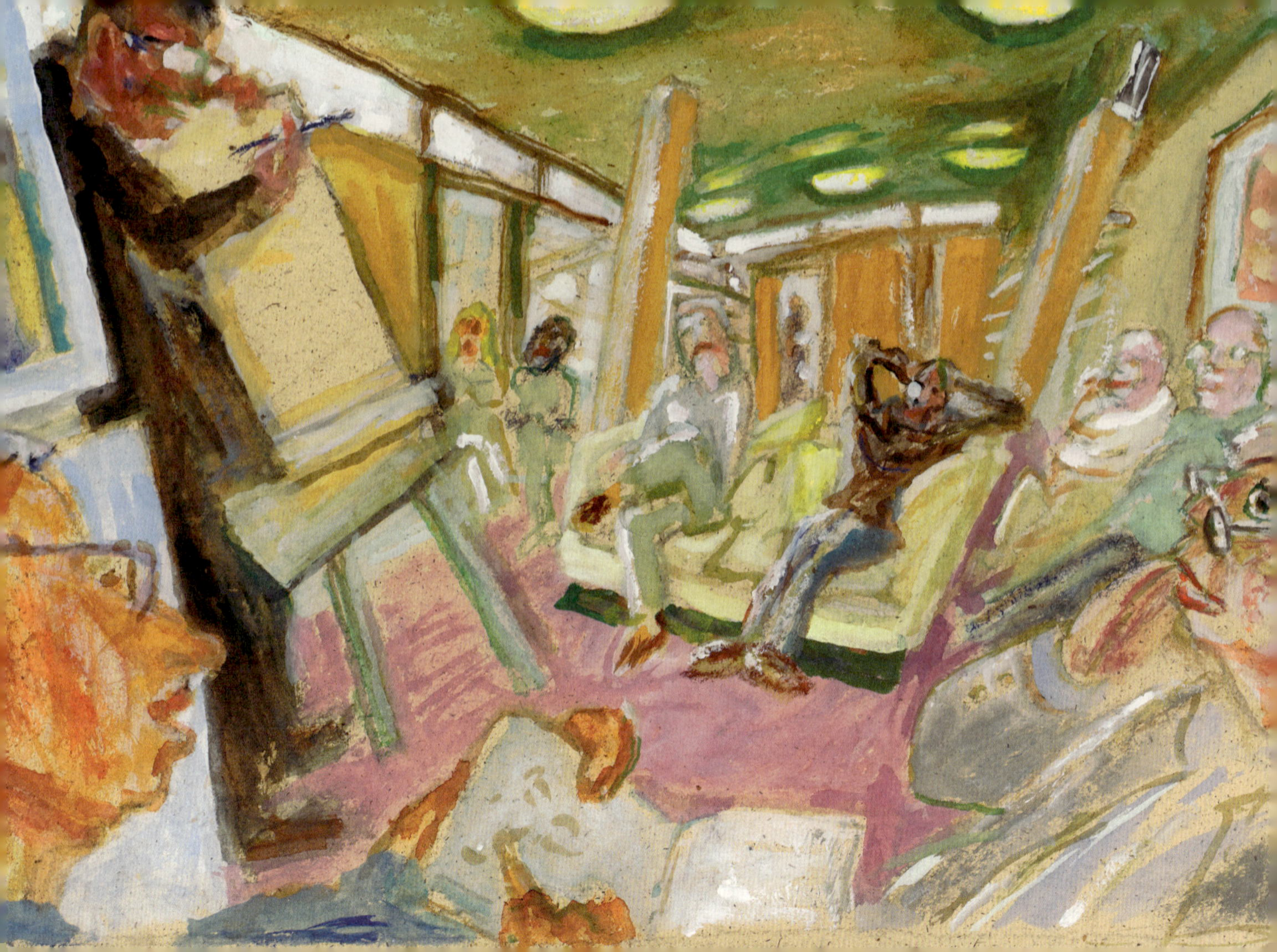

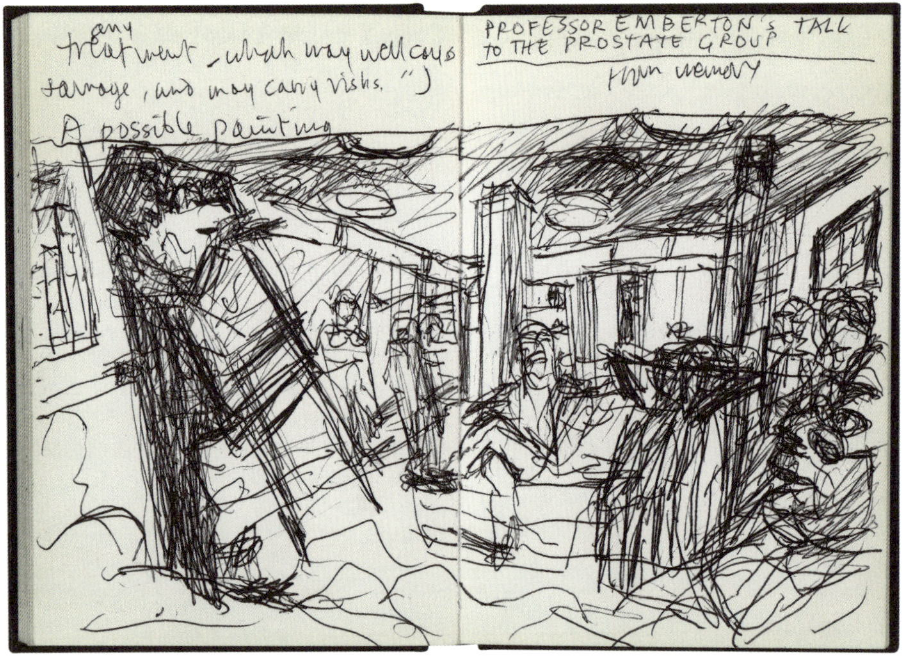
any
treatment, which may well cause
damage, and may carry risks.")
A possible painting
PROFESSOR EMBERTON'S TALK
TO THE PROSTATE GROUP
from memory

*Mark Emberton Talks to the Prostate Group II*

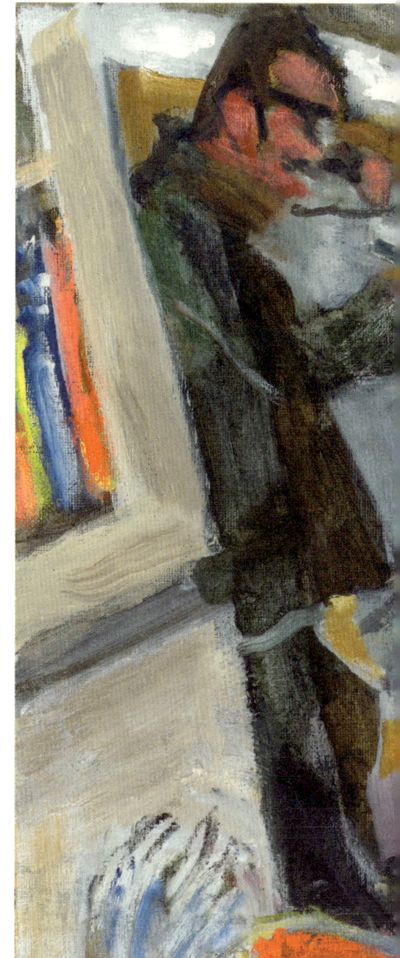

*Mark Emberton Talks to the Prostate Group III*

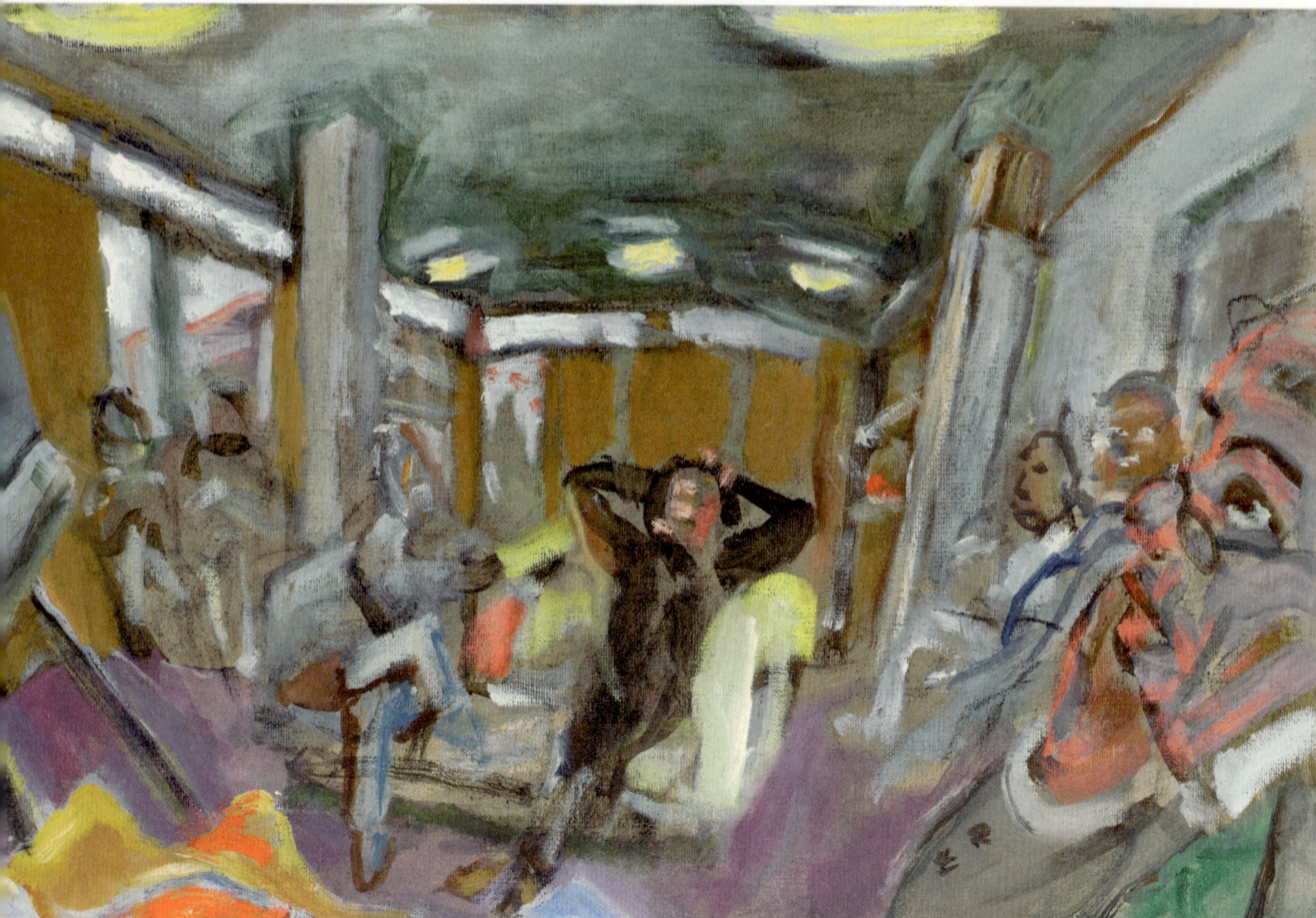

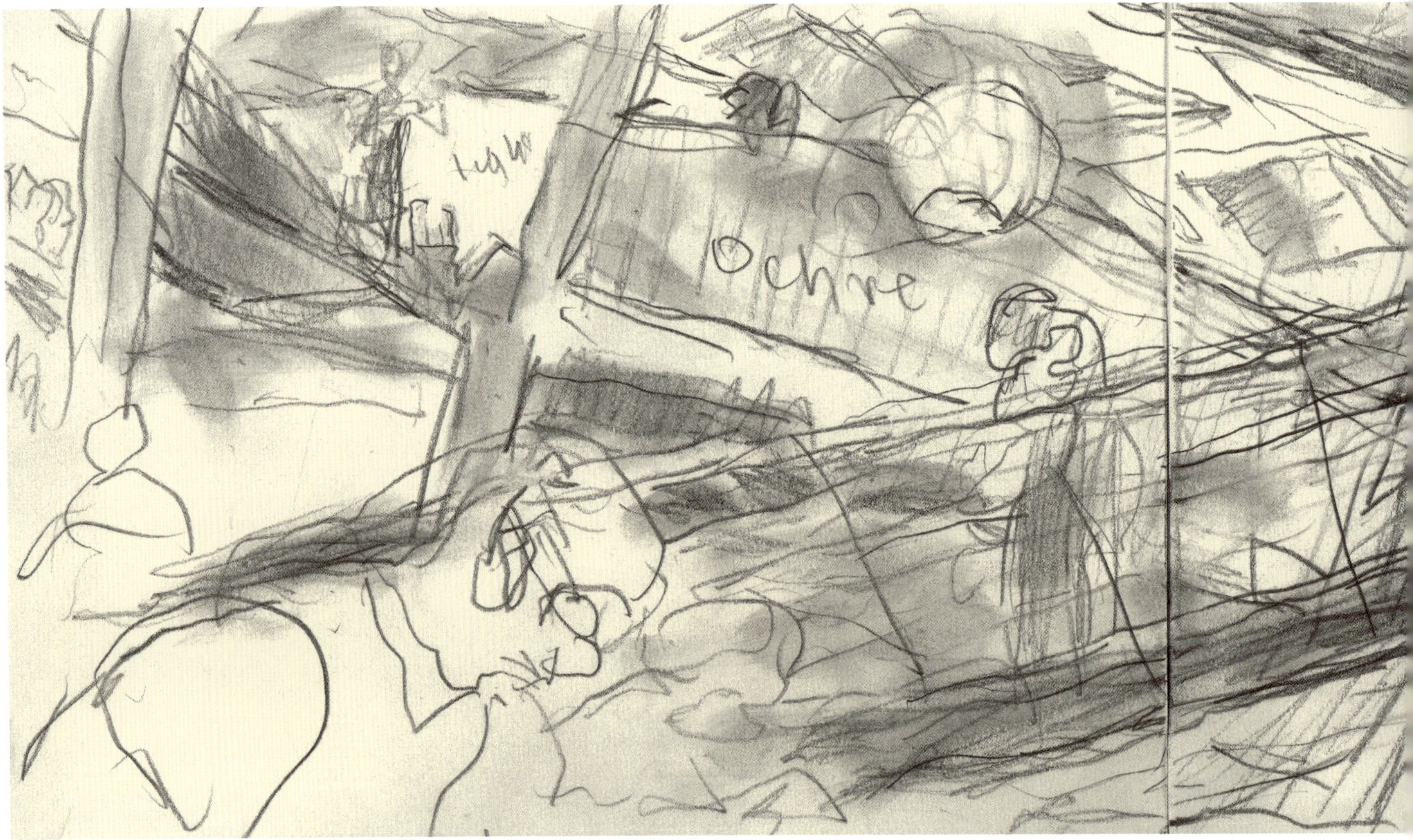
Ochre

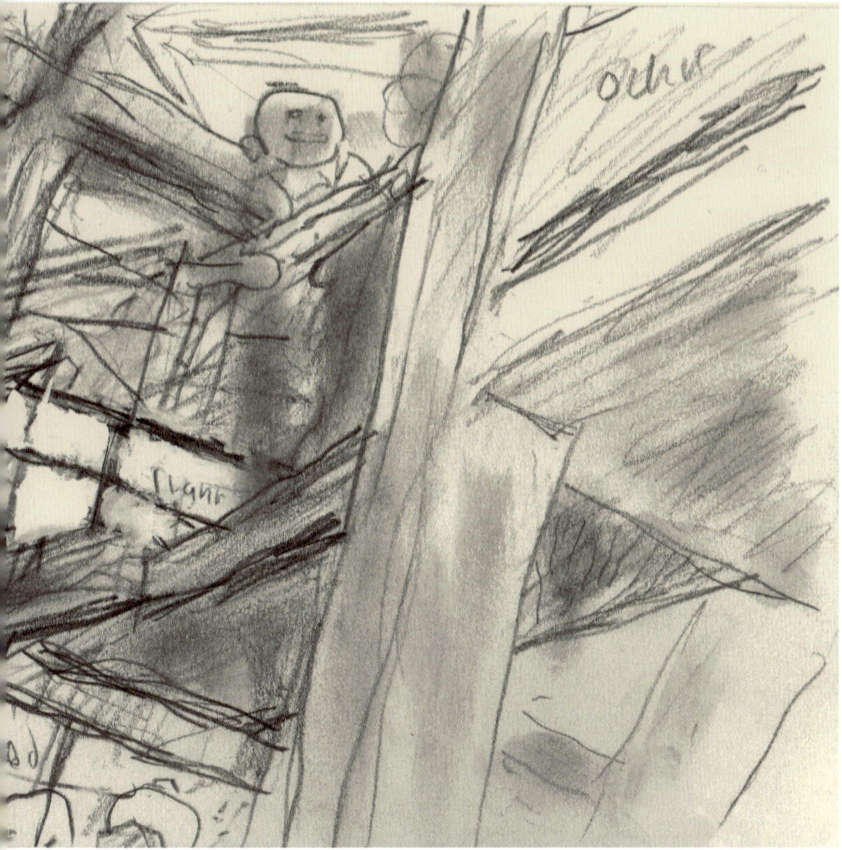

*Tuesday 24 April*
Arriving at about 12.30 pm, I immediately run into E, who is looking a lot better. I draw her waiting for the relaxation class to begin. When it does, I stay put, taking my place at the table, but with my back to the window, facing the stairs, trying just to enjoy the passage of people.

*With My Back to the Window*

## MAY 2012

*Tuesday 1 May*

I have arranged to draw Y, who came in looking stricken. I persuade her to start drawing, and she does very well in the little sketchbook I lend her – intent, searching – much better than me! My own drawings remain chaotic, ugly. Yet there may be the germ of a picture here – perhaps a gouache? Later I see E, as well as Nicholas, Marjorie, Nigel. I also speak with a stranger beside me, who is suffering from Bell's palsy as well as cancer, and she says she finds the informality of Maggie's a bit disconcerting.

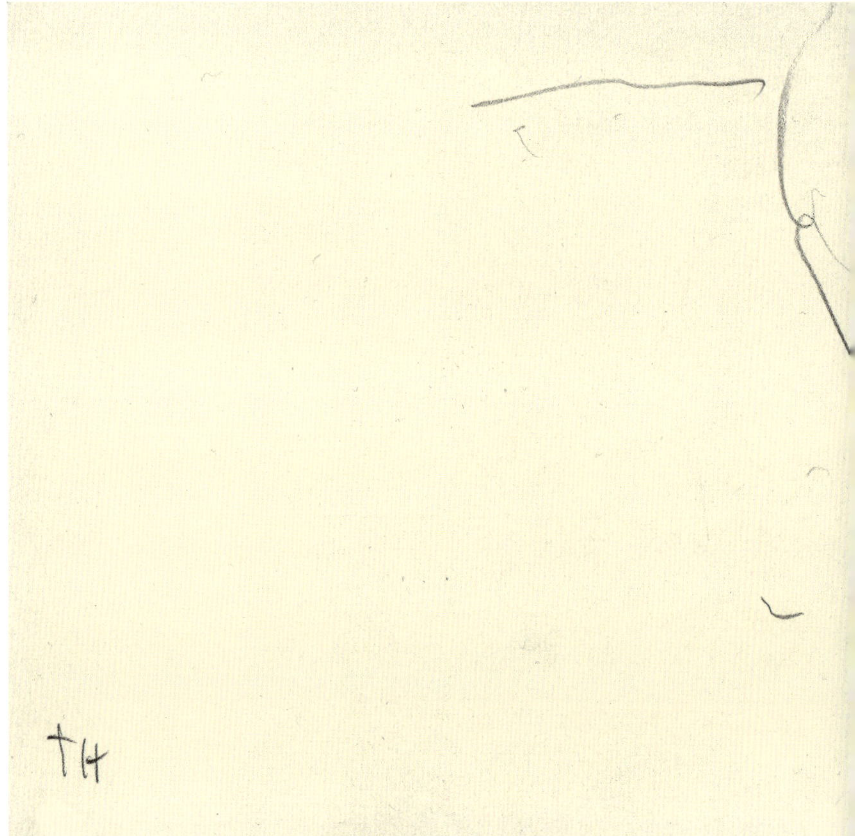

*Y Looking Stricken*

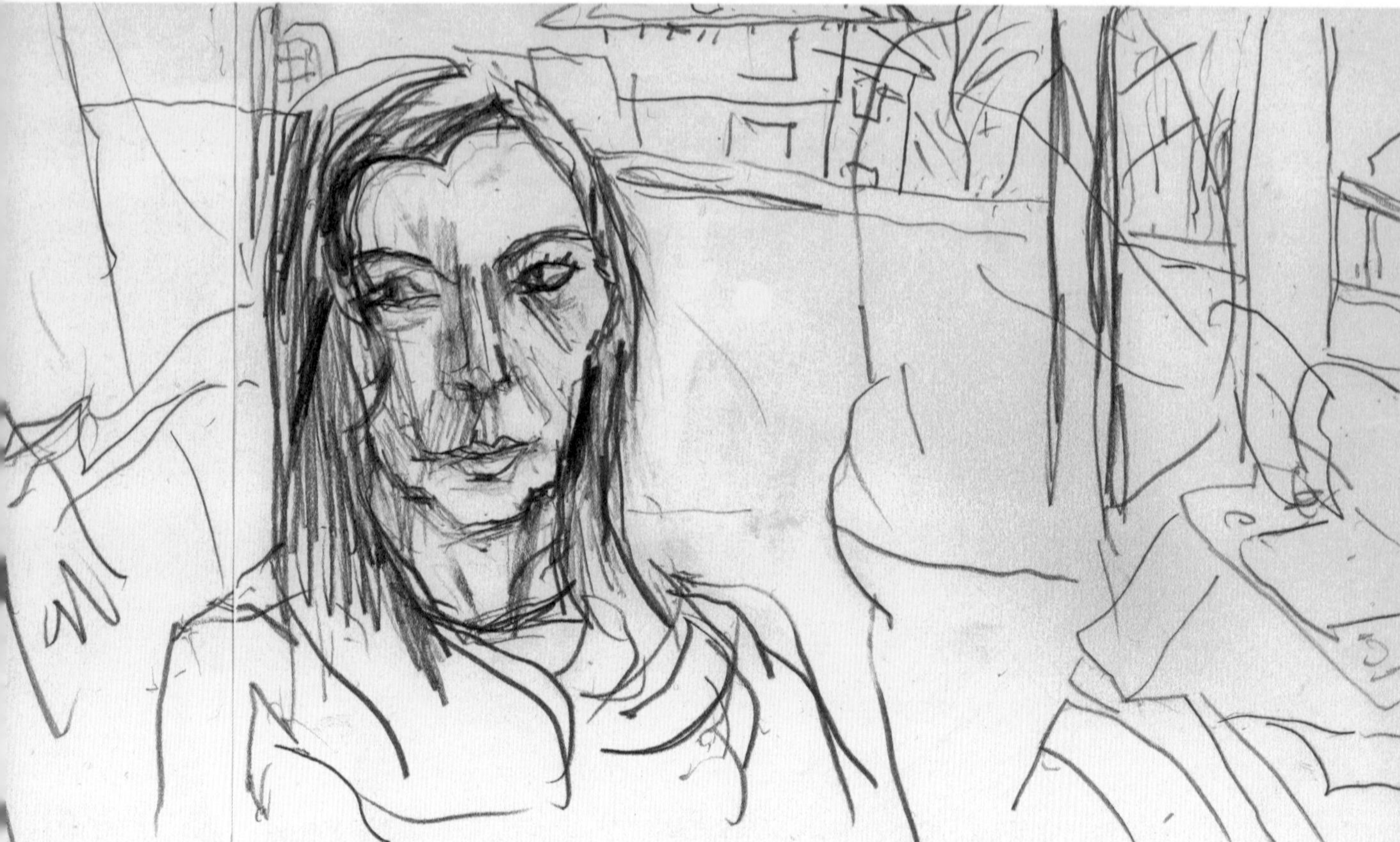

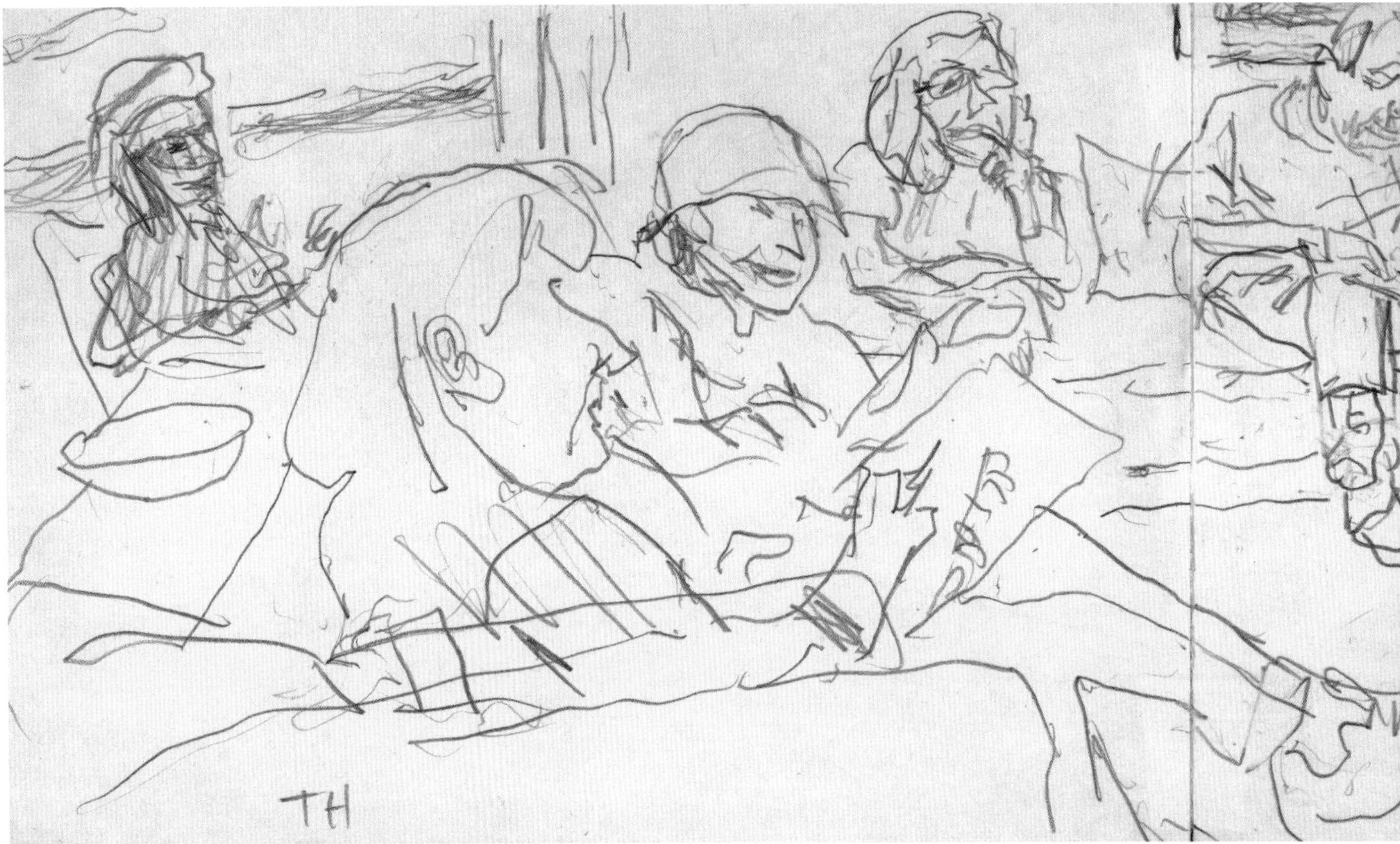


*Nutrition I*

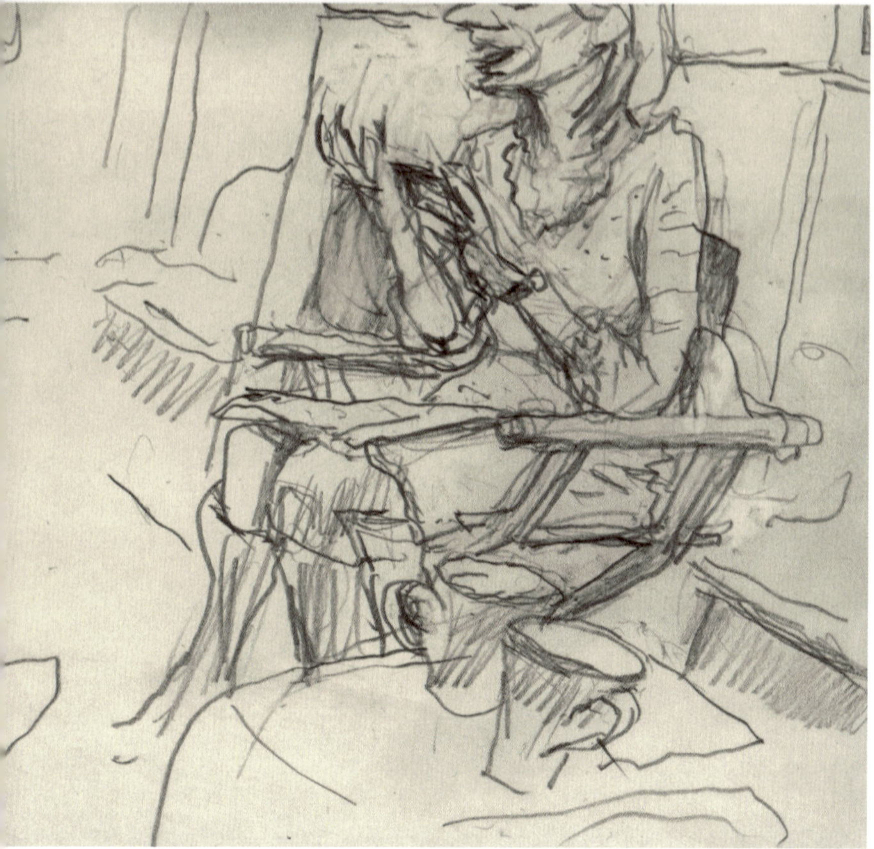

*Monday 14 May*
Today it's the Nutrition Class, which has rather a chaotic beginning, with only five participants at first; another seven eventually drift in. I'm not drawing well. But from noon I'm with the Prostate Group again and I do better. One treatment is defined as 'chemical castration'. And several members of the group complain about an unexpected consequence of surgery that no one had warned them about: a kind of nip-and-tuck that results in your losing two inches of penis length!

OVERLEAF *Nutrition II*

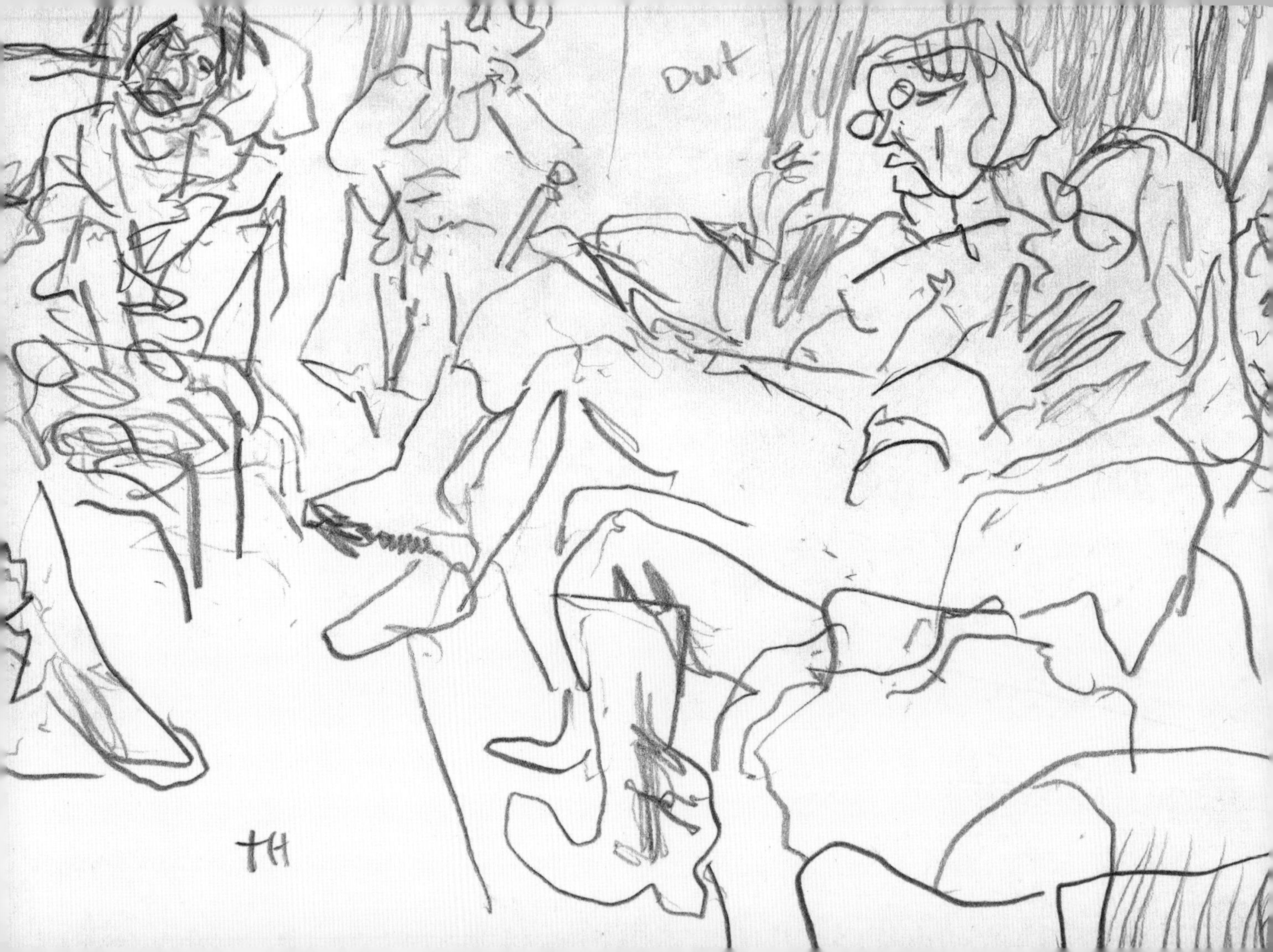
Dut
TH

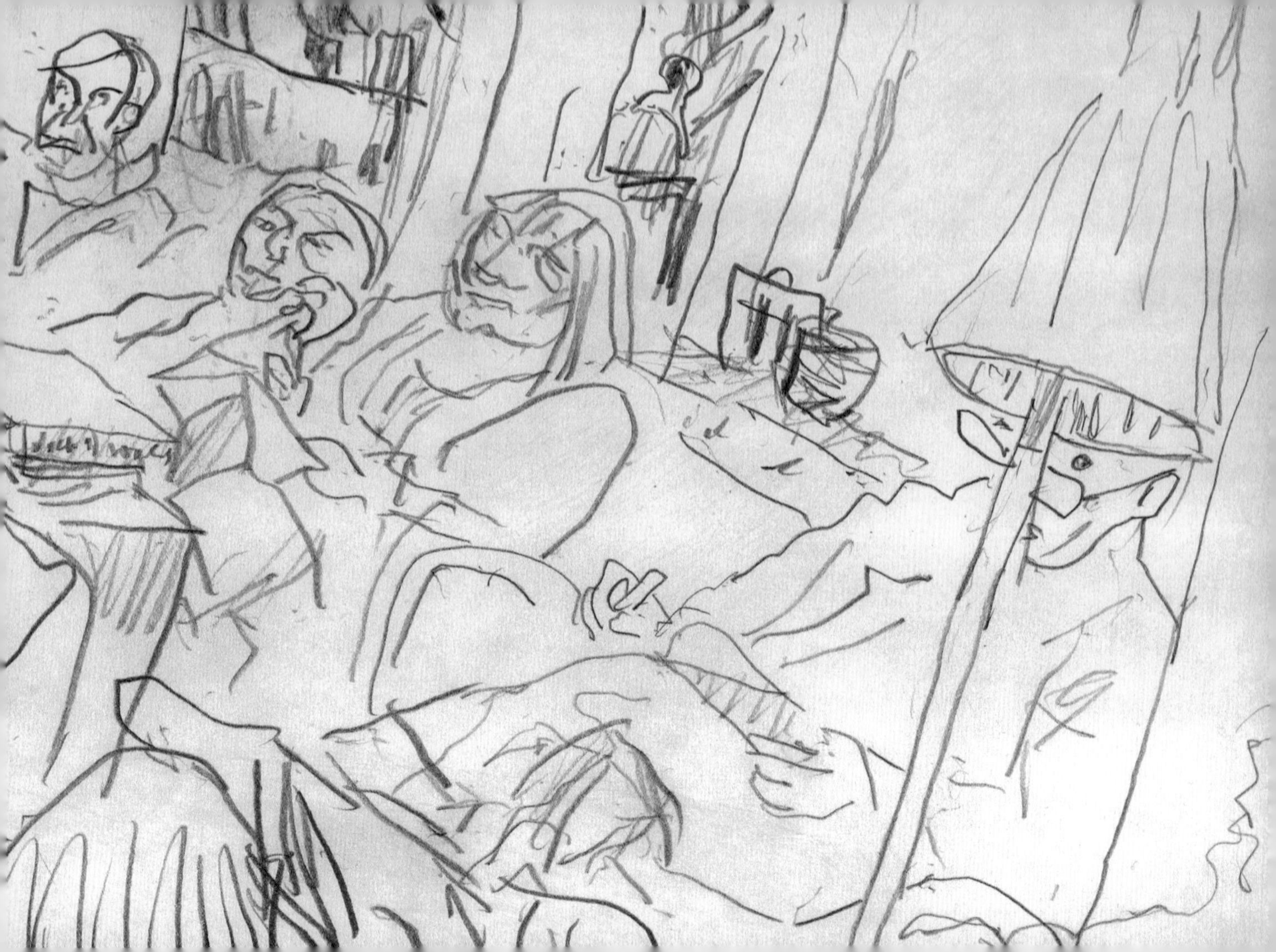

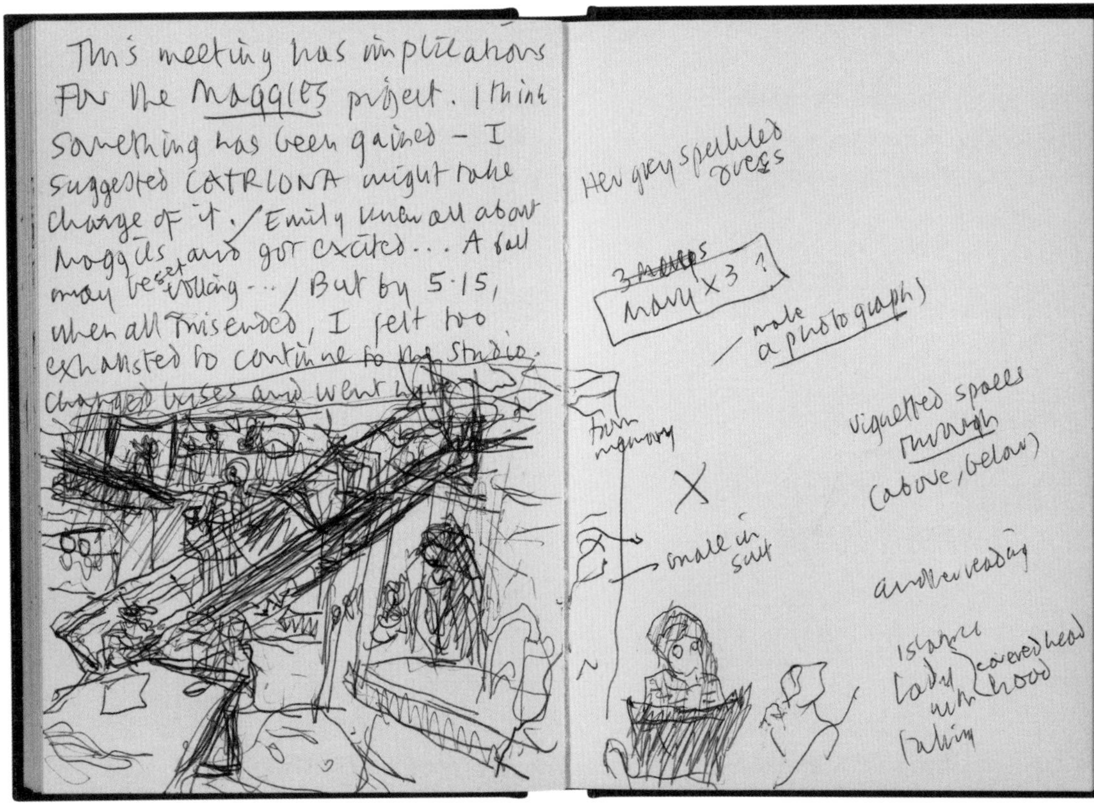
This meeting has implications
for the MAGGIES project. I think
something has been gained – I
suggested CATRIONA might take
charge of it. / Emily knew all about
Maggies and got excited... A ball
may be set rolling... / But by 5.15,
when all this ended, I felt too
exhausted to continue to the studio.
Changed buses and went home
Her grey speckled dress
Mary x 3 ?
make a photograph
from memory
snake in suit
vignetted spaces through
(above, below)
another reading
Islamic lady covered head with hood
talking

*Wednesday 23 May*
I draw Bernie, hunched with concern as she bends towards someone at the table. Back at home I sort my drawings for Richard Cork's visit (he's writing a piece on my residency for *RA Magazine*). Sometimes the most presentable are not the most interesting; the wilder ones have their place too.

*Tuesday 29 May*
I am tired after yesterday's Varnishing Day at the RA. After lunch I just keep the pencil moving around the peopled space, rather enjoyably: spaces too complex to represent, one could say. My images are made up of glimpses, with all sorts of figures floating about at the margins.

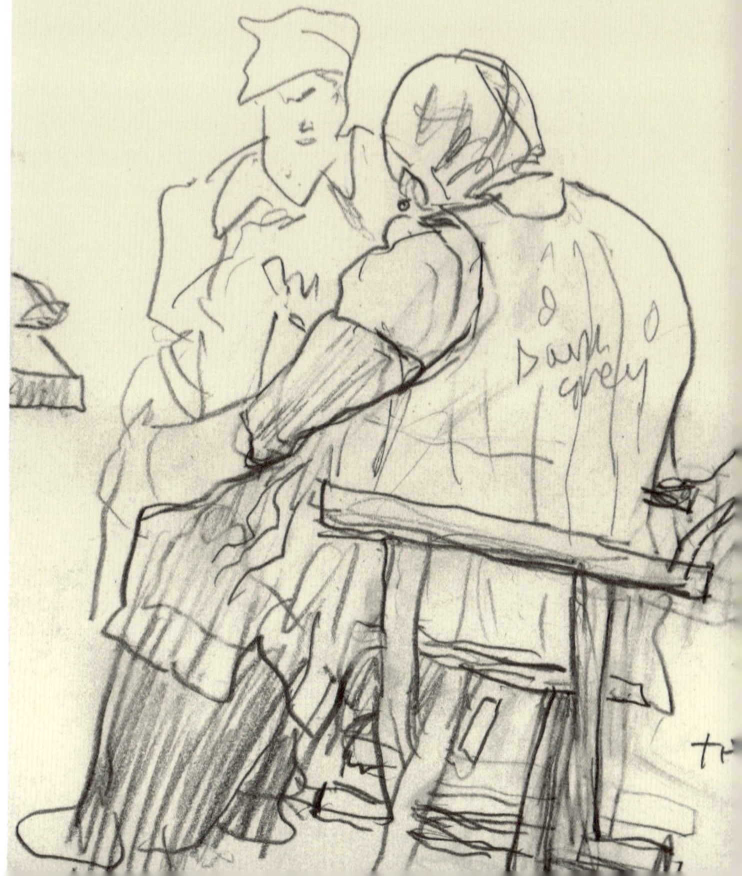


*Bernie*

## JUNE 2012

*Wednesday 6 June*

I embark on a long-arranged expedition to Scotland, heartland of Maggie's. First to Glasgow. Set just below the huge hilltop towers of the University, the Gatehouse appears tiny, almost negligible; but inside one finds it very cannily converted by the architects Page & Park, who have packed in a large variety of possible spaces and combinations. (It is more homely, and warmer than 'my' Maggie's in London.) As Stuart Danskin, the Cancer Support Specialist, explains, 'West-of-Scotland Man has confounded our expectations'; 45% of users here are male. There are several different levels: up from the kitchen to the handsome sitting room with its stove (which at first I mistake for a television) and well-upholstered armchairs and sofa, and then beyond, the larger space, with an aquarium, and even stuffed animals. Marie McQuade, Maggie's Development Director (Culture and Innovation), meets me, nursing her baby, and I feel immediately on her wavelength. We have a frank talk about the 'real' content of what happens at Maggie's. She says, unbidden, 'AN EXISTENTIAL CRISIS'. Exactly! Then I move into the Fish Room, where the Prostate Group is meeting. These men look like members of the same family – heavily built, bald, with specs, genial and friendly. It is all very informal; they are just chatting away, with much laughter, probably not very much about cancer. After I've drawn for a while, an elder joins me. He tells me only eight have died out of 140 in the nine years he's been coming to the group. I enjoy their animation, the sense of a flourishing social exchange – and the fish in between.

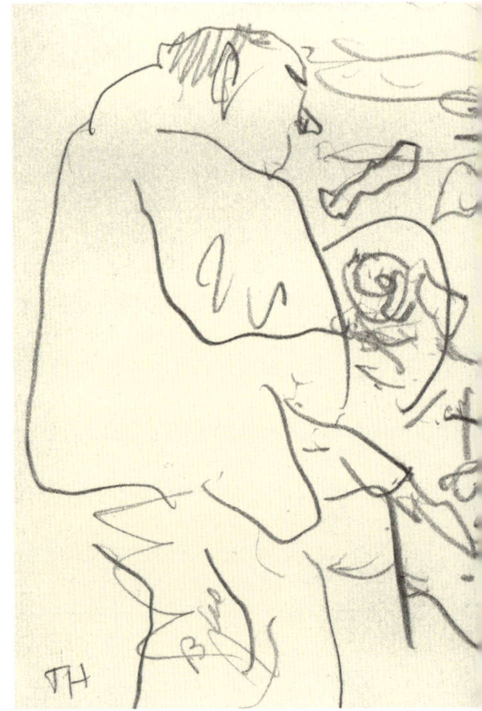

*At Glasgow Gatehouse: The Fish Room I*

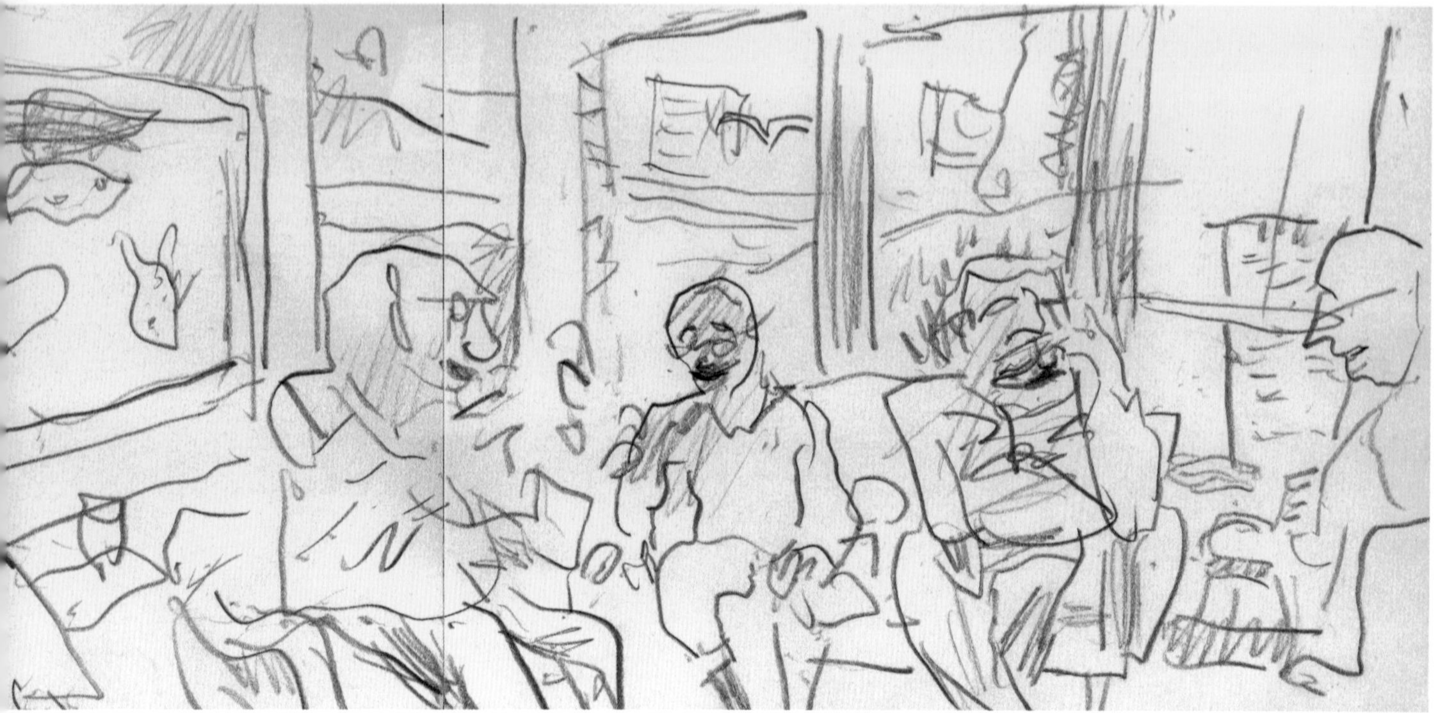

OVERLEAF *At Glasgow Gatehouse: The Fish Room II*

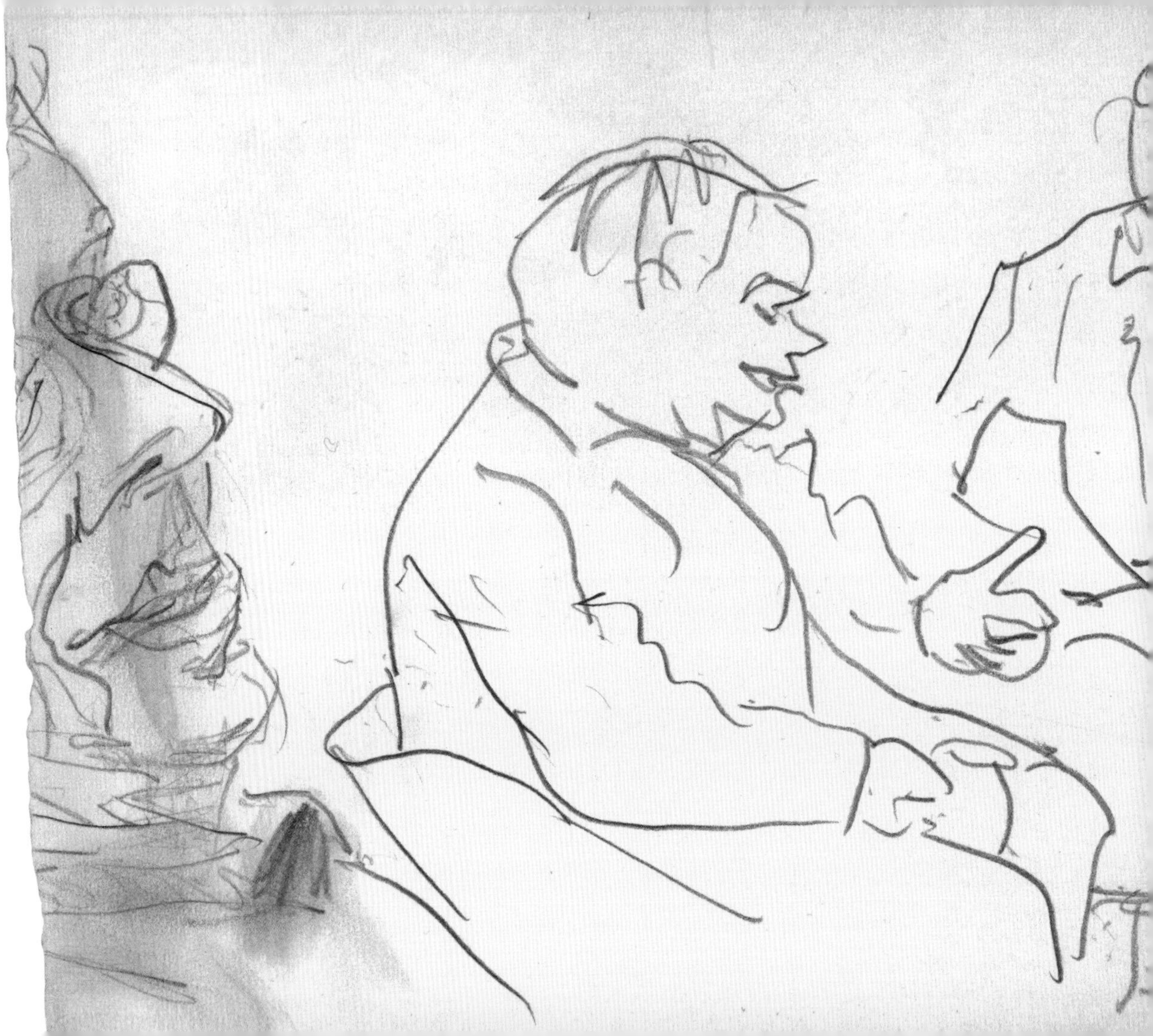

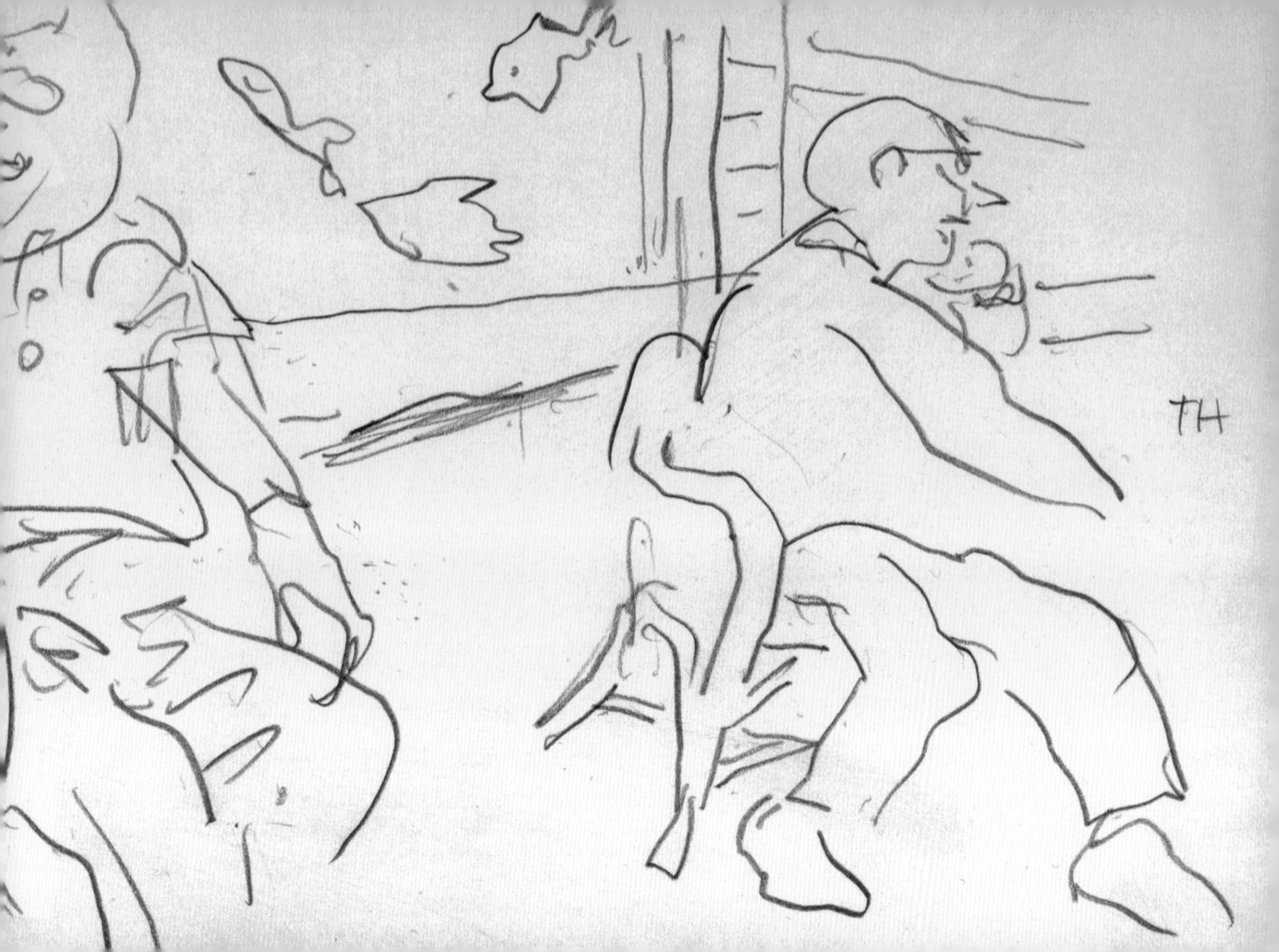
TH

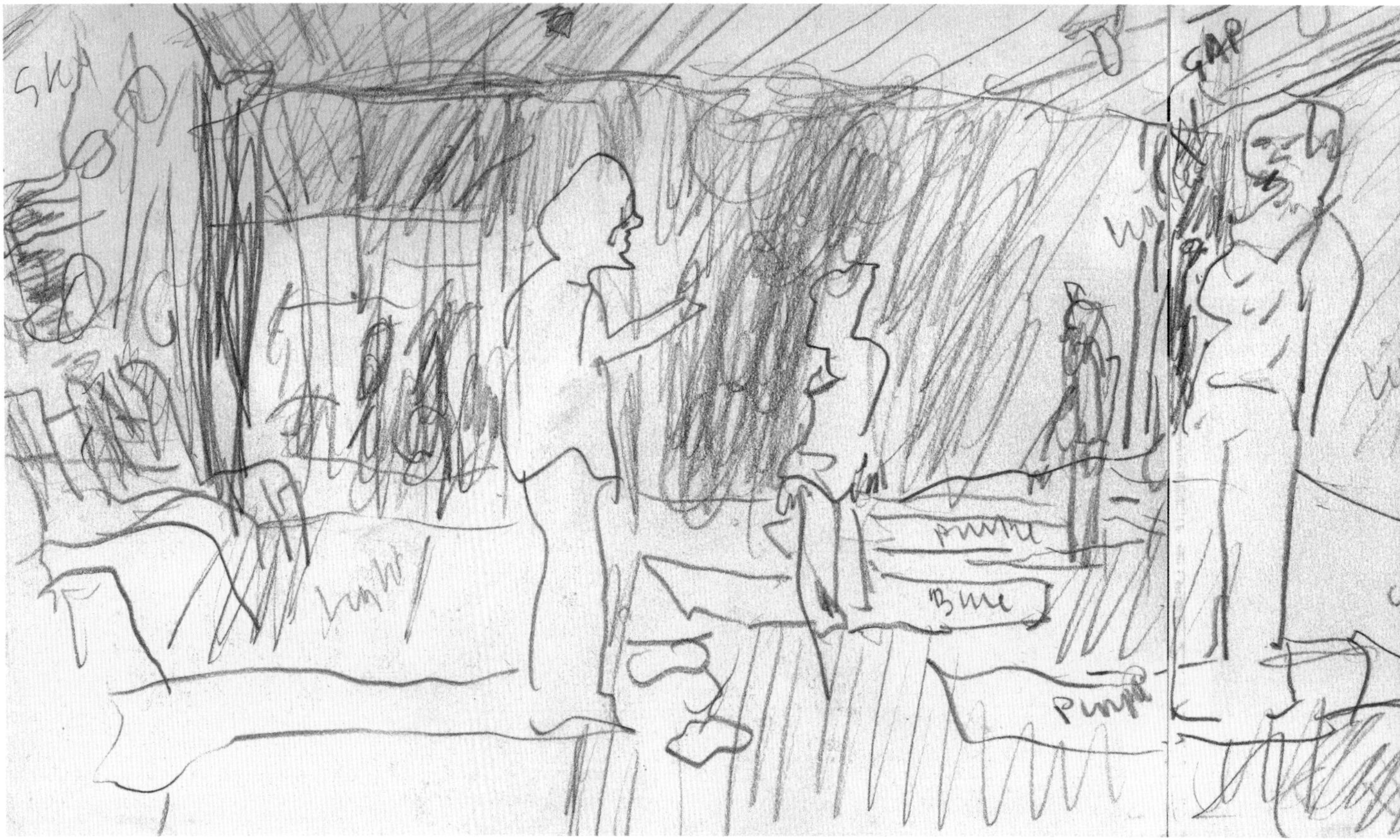


*The Yoga Class at Gartnavel I*

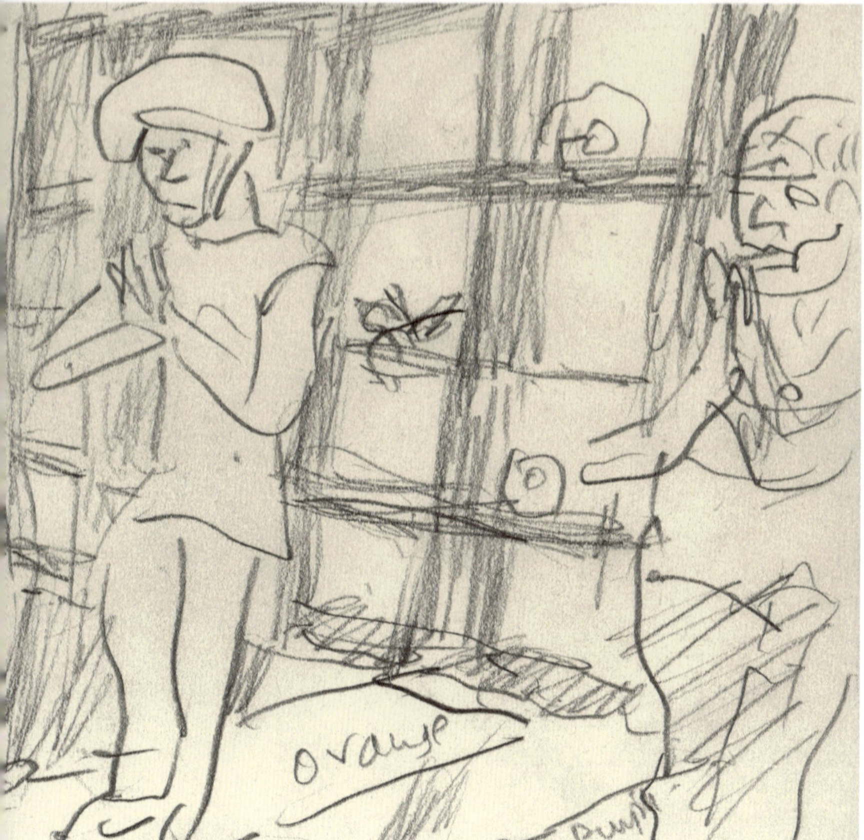


In the afternoon I arrive at Gartnavel Hospital in Glasgow, where the Maggie's Centre by Rem Koolhaas has recently opened. After the Gatehouse, it feels very 'Euro' – a child of, say, the Louisiana Museum outside Copenhagen. A bit sterile? There's lots of wooden shelving, and compartments for designer items. In a wooden, sauna-like room, there are fleeces on the benches, but it is mostly continuous corridor, of which the offices are a part – a doughnut around a green core planted by Maggie's daughter Lily. It is a very intelligent architecture and does create a flow of space. In the yoga class the female instructor, something of a guru, has taught for forty years. She moves beautifully, conveying a sense of both body and spirit. The mats are orange, purple, pale blue.

OVERLEAF *The Yoga Class at Gartnavel II*

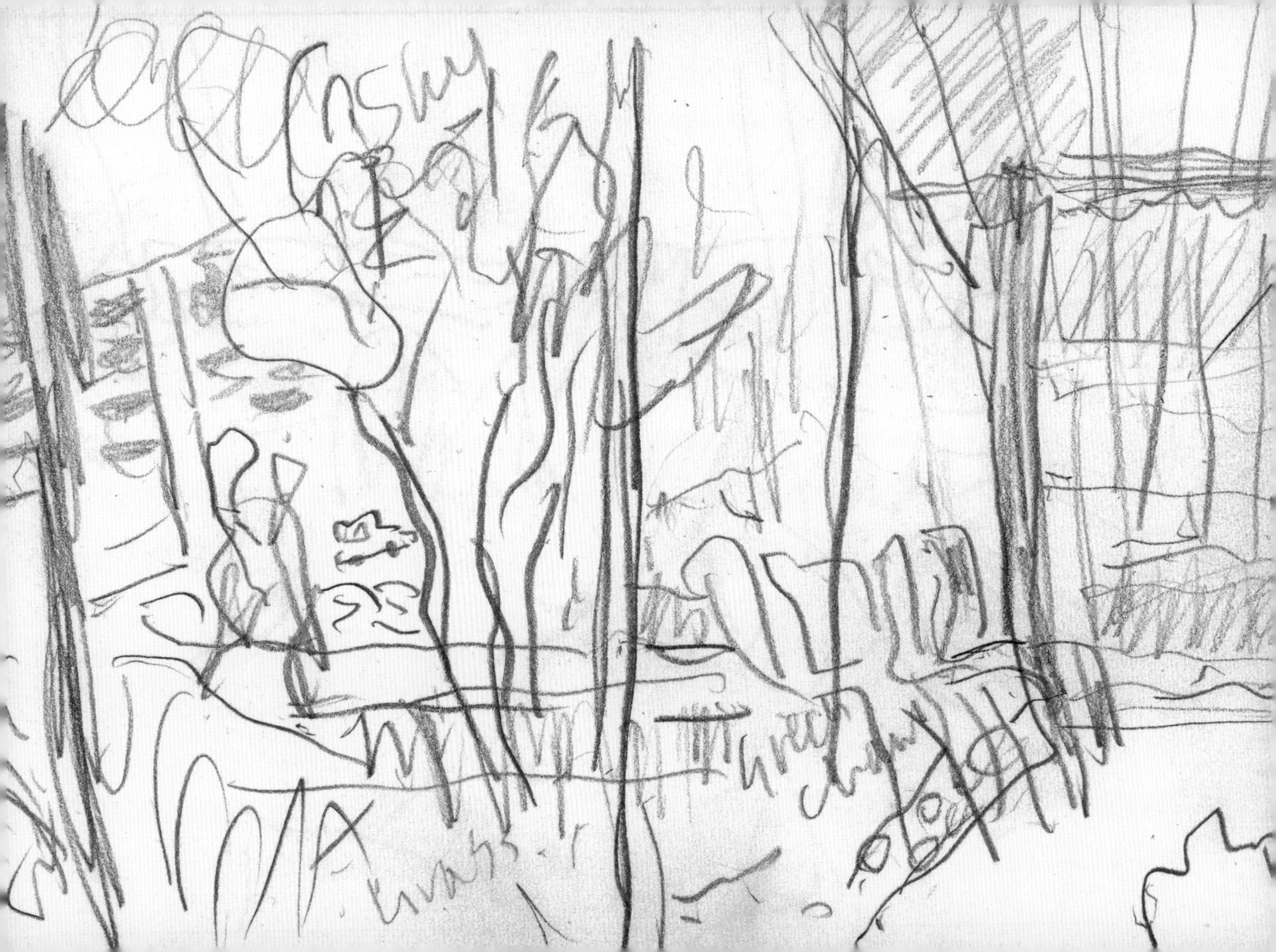
grass

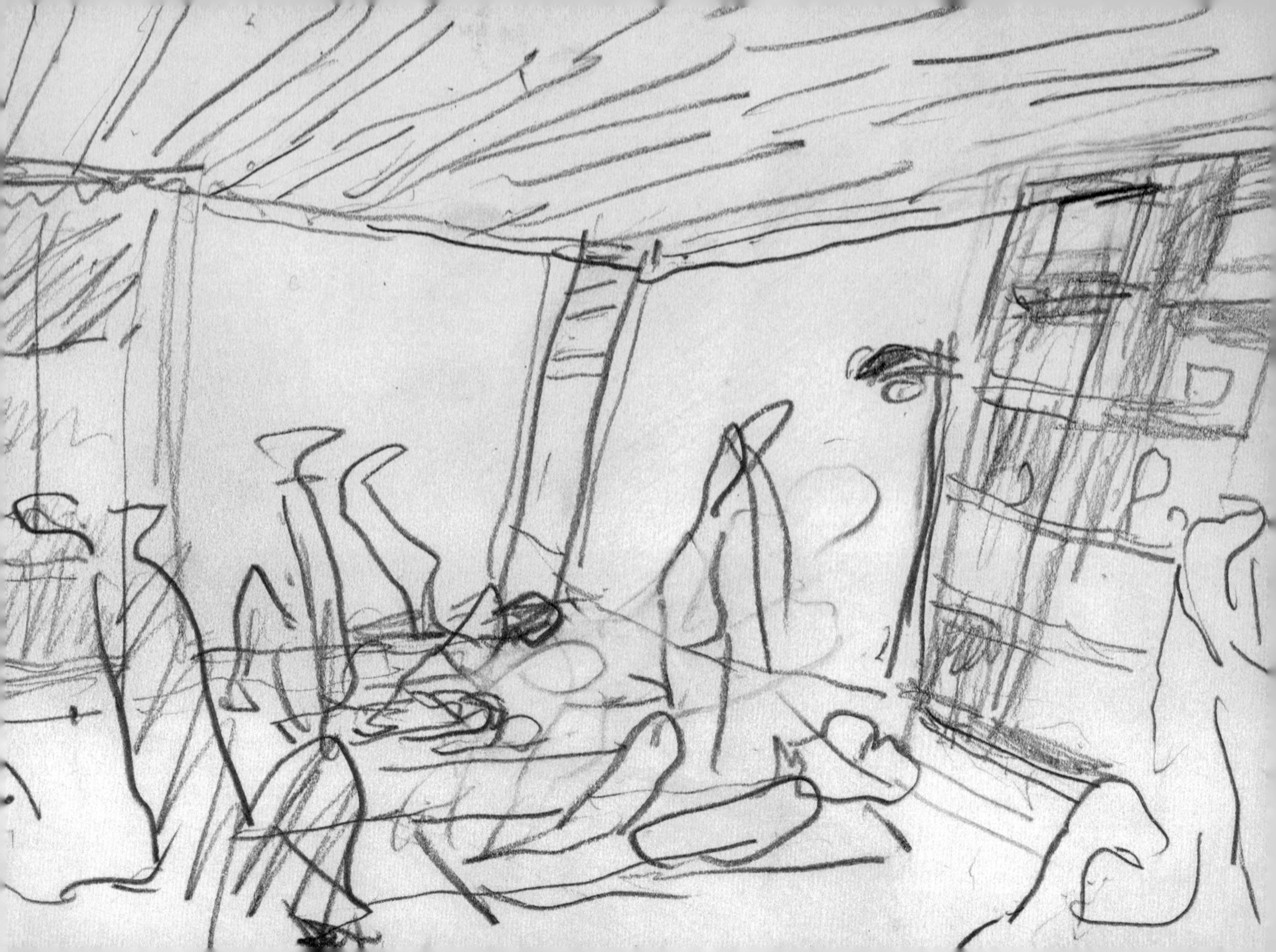

*Thursday 7 June*
I move on to Edinburgh, where I will be staying with an old painting comrade, Sandy Moffat, former Head of Painting at Glasgow School of Art. We meet at Waverley Station for the beautiful train journey together out to Dundee, where Frank Gehry built perhaps the most famous of the Maggie's Centres so far.

I sit in blessed sun above the 'silvery Tay' and make both a pencil drawing and a pastel. Gehry's is a marvellous building – a small wonder-of-the-world, a joyful event-in-the-landscape. Sandy and I both see it as a *metaphorical* building: we swap 'associations' – of a windmill, of Sydney Opera House, an African hut or a prehistoric broch, Le Corbusier's Ronchamp or Rudolf Steiner's Goetheanum, a lighthouse, a Swiss chalet, an aeroplane… (the site was originally the hospital's helipad). Afterwards I feel ready to descend and make more human contact. We settle around the table. Behind us, two people are talking on the beautiful little wooden platform jettied out from the hill. We talk about the documentary film that has just been completed here, *Tuesdays*, made by Amy Hardie, sister of the painter Gwen, both of them well known to Sandy. He is becoming a huge enthusiast for Maggie's now.

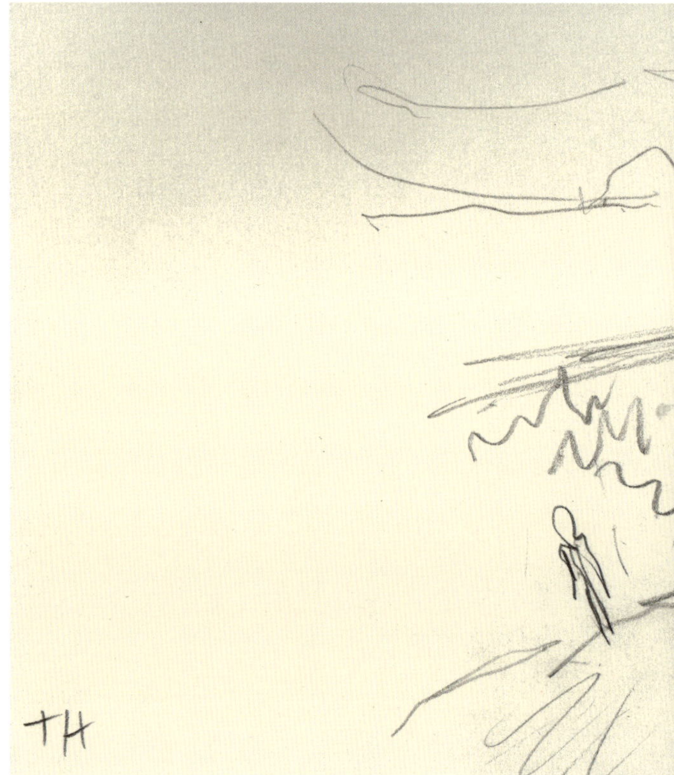

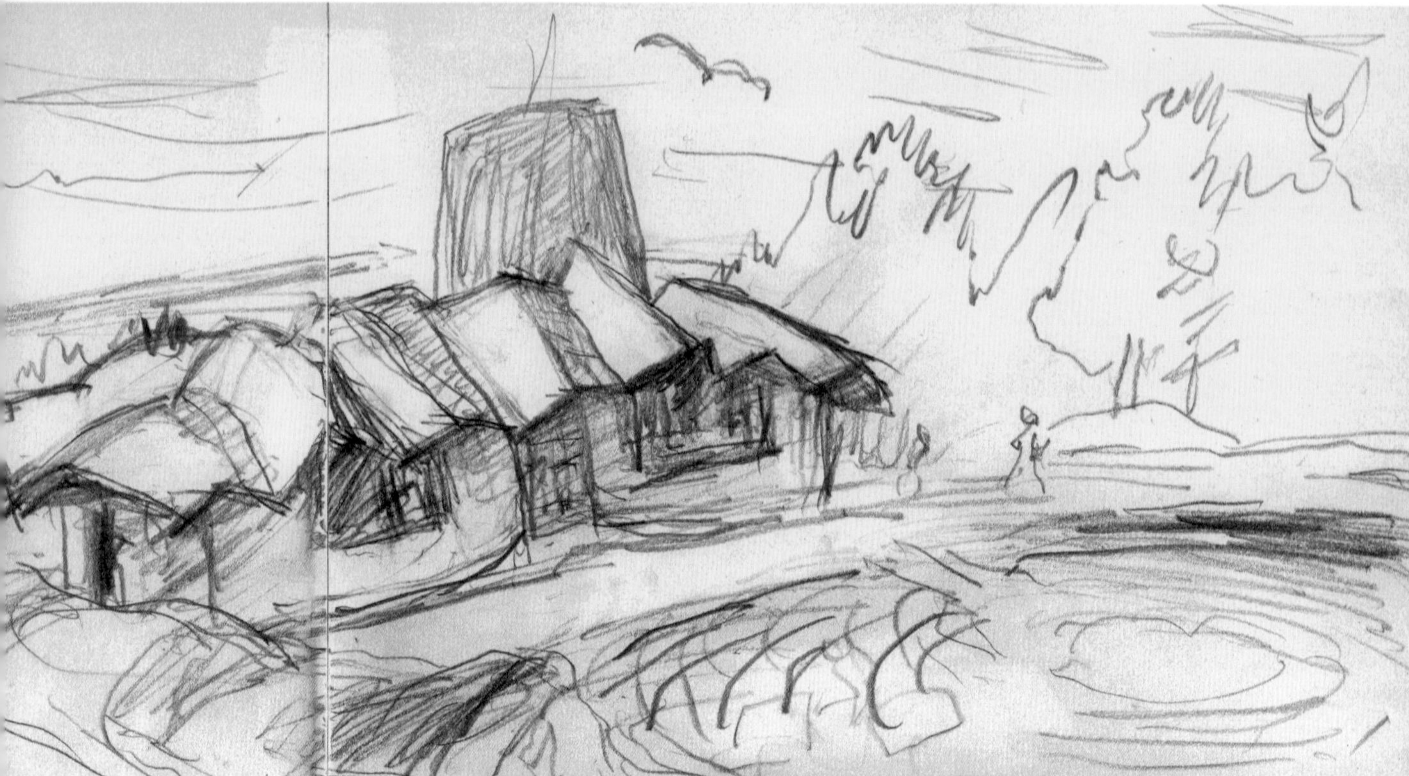

*Gehry's Broch, Dundee*

OVERLEAF *The Prostate Group V*

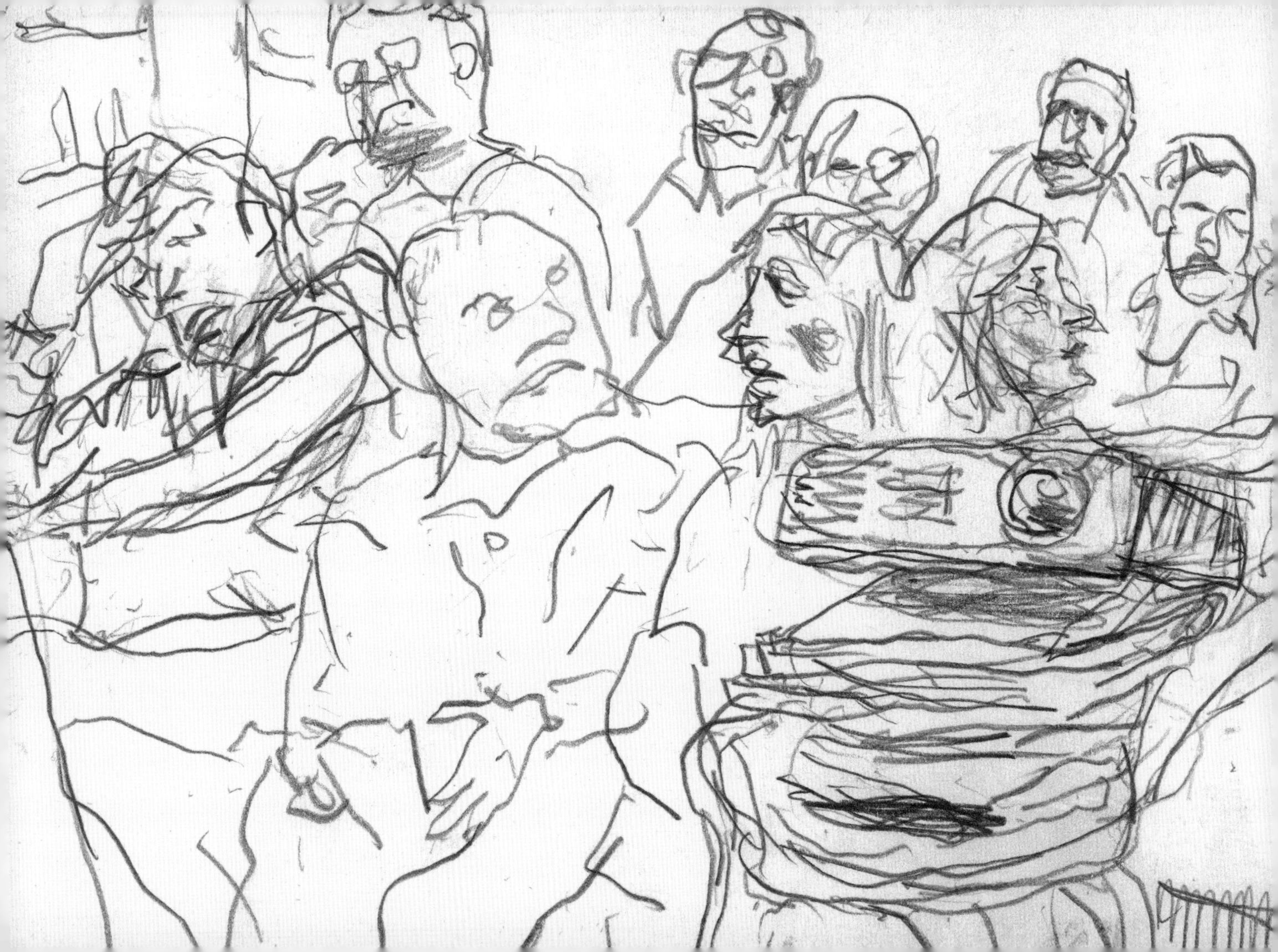

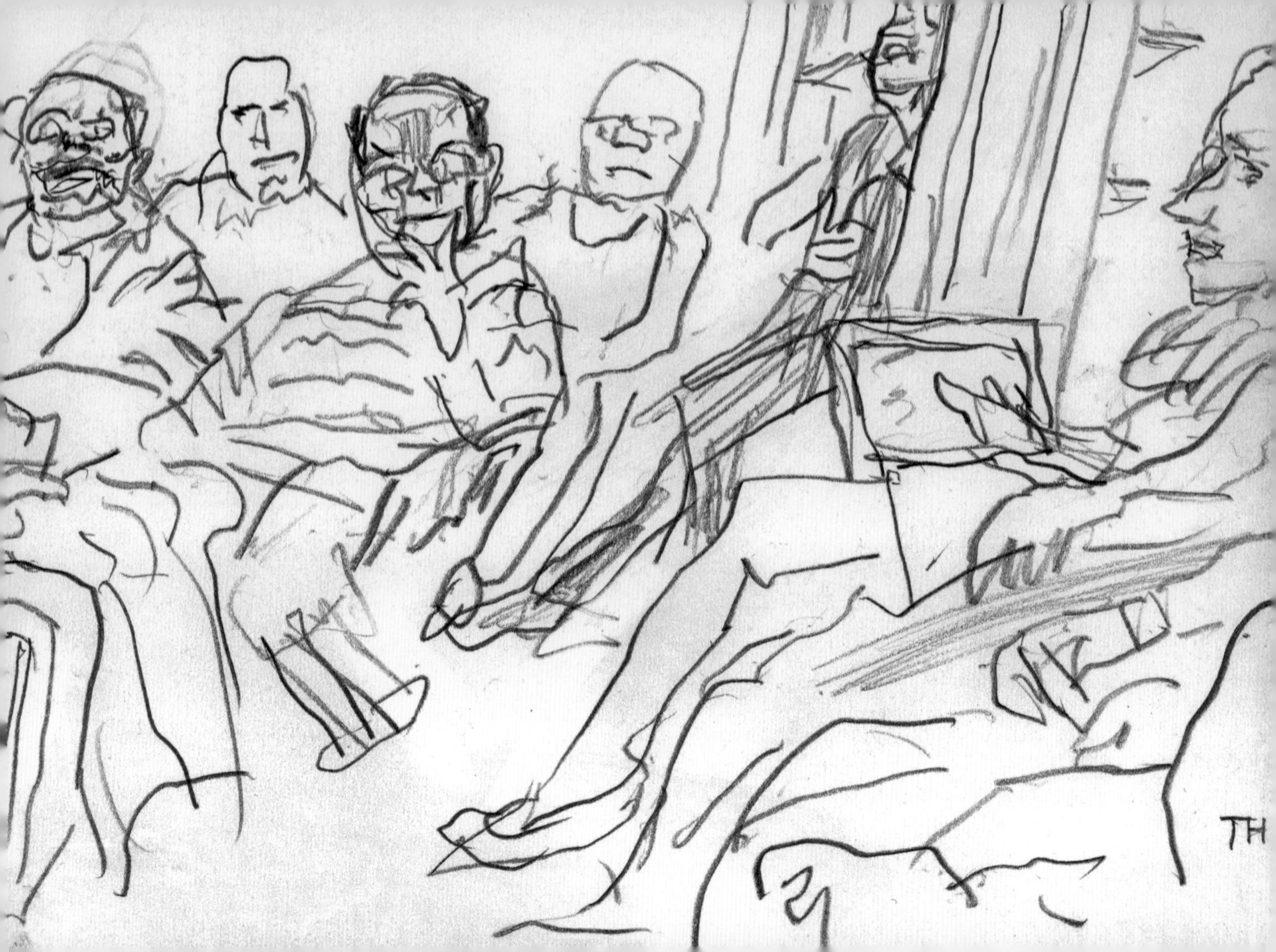
TH

*Friday 8 June*
Still with Sandy, I visit the original Maggie's, the little mothership, beside the Western General Hospital in Edinburgh, a stables converted by Richard Murphy Architects. The Gehry building we saw yesterday is a hard act to follow, but in its modest way the Edinburgh centre is very user-friendly. A bright place, even in this drizzly haar – full of colour, variations of pinks and lime greens.

*Monday 15 June*
Back in London, I once again join the Prostate Group at 'my' Maggie's. Two female nurses talk to us males about the practicalities of incontinence; the devices that can be fitted, the exercises.

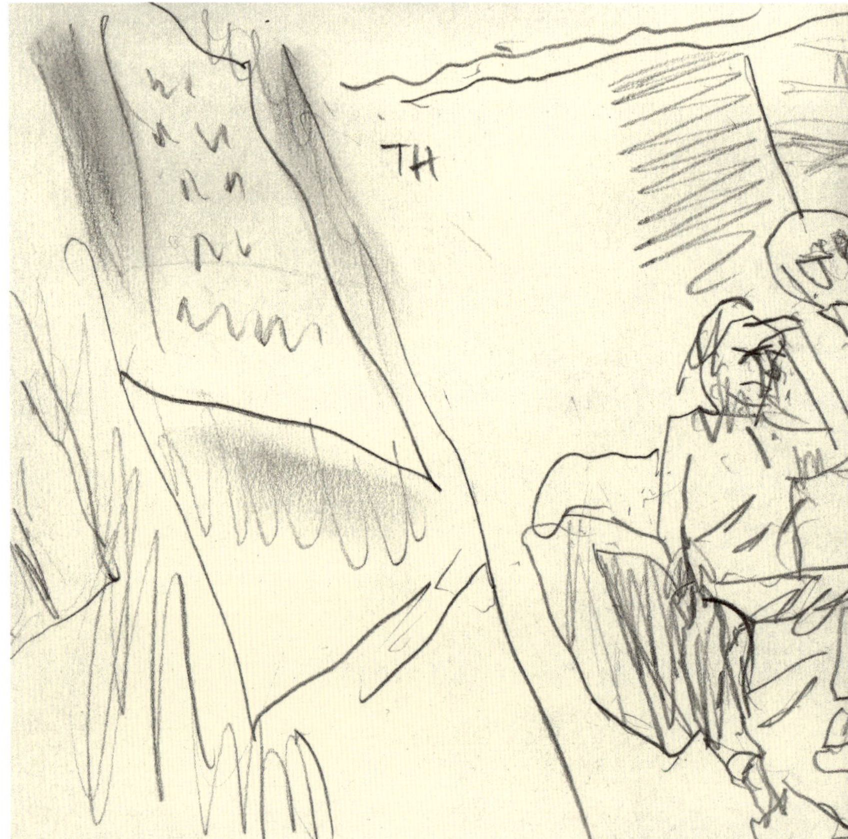

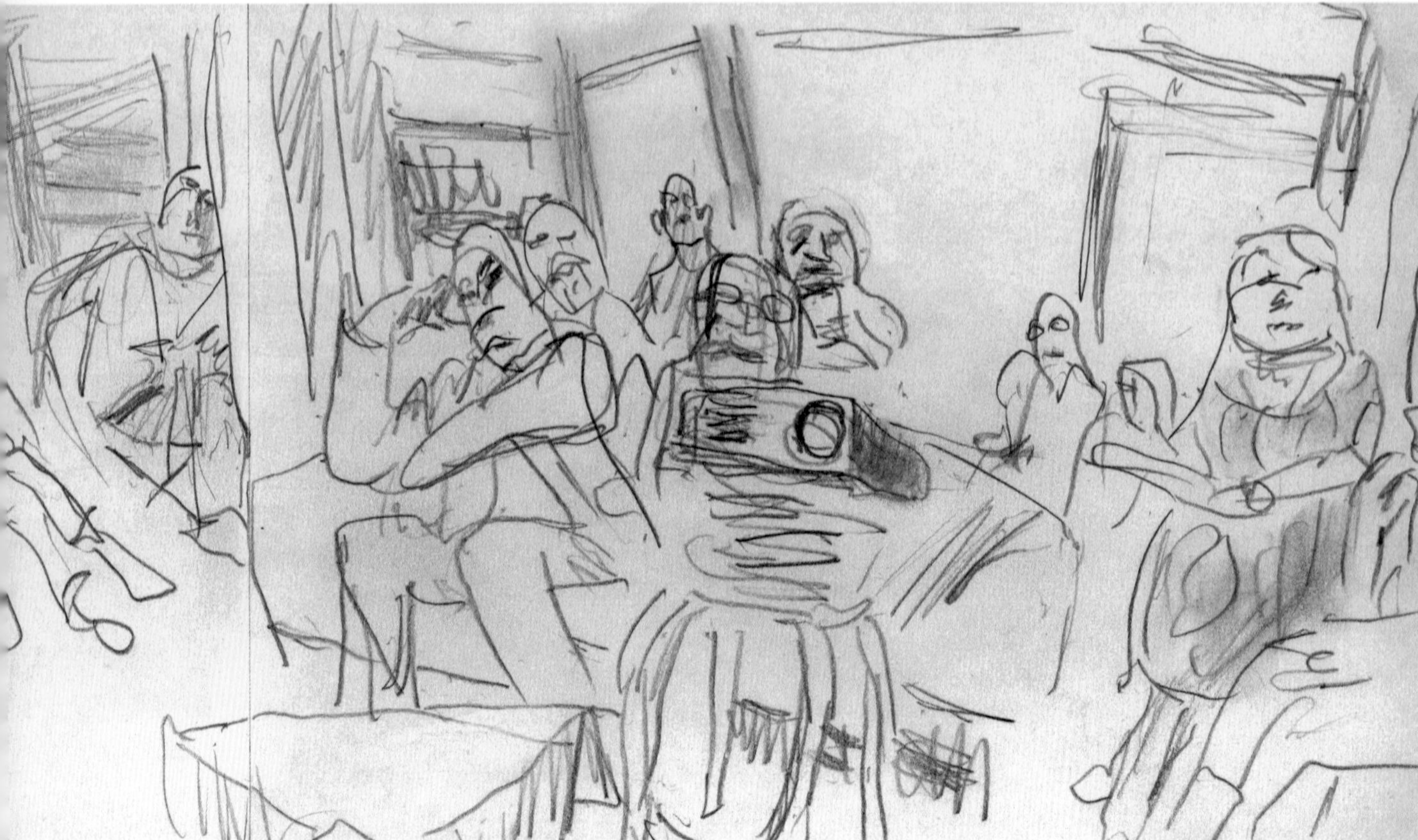

*The Prostate Group VI*

*Thursday 21 June*
I meet up with Philipp Ebeling, the photographer for Richard Cork's *RA Magazine* article. After a grey start there are shafts of sunlight. Philipp photographs me drawing, then we rope in E, who does seem a much happier person. (Touchingly, she says the drawing sessions have made a real difference to her relationship with Maggie's.) I then have a surprising drawing session at the table: a beautiful young black woman, completely bald, talks to the nurse as her white partner looks on. She is living at Charing Cross Hospital while undergoing an intensive course of chemotherapy.

Various ideas are discussed. For example, I might 'shadow' Jay, when he discusses benefits. Draw as a fly-on-the-wall in some one-to-one sessions, or perhaps join the Young Men's Group? In practice, none of these proves possible, either because the users' group responds negatively, or because I can't get there on the right day.

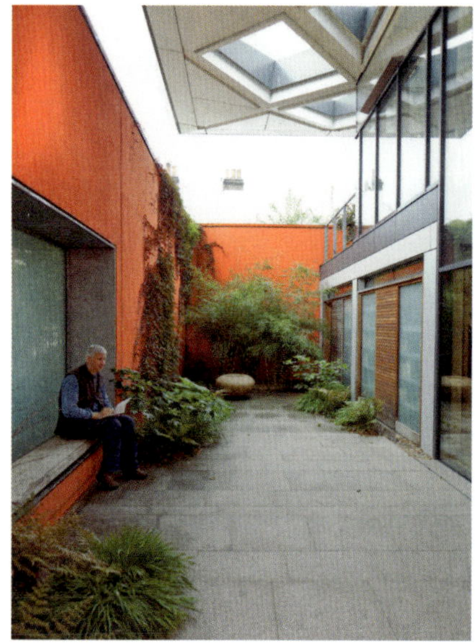

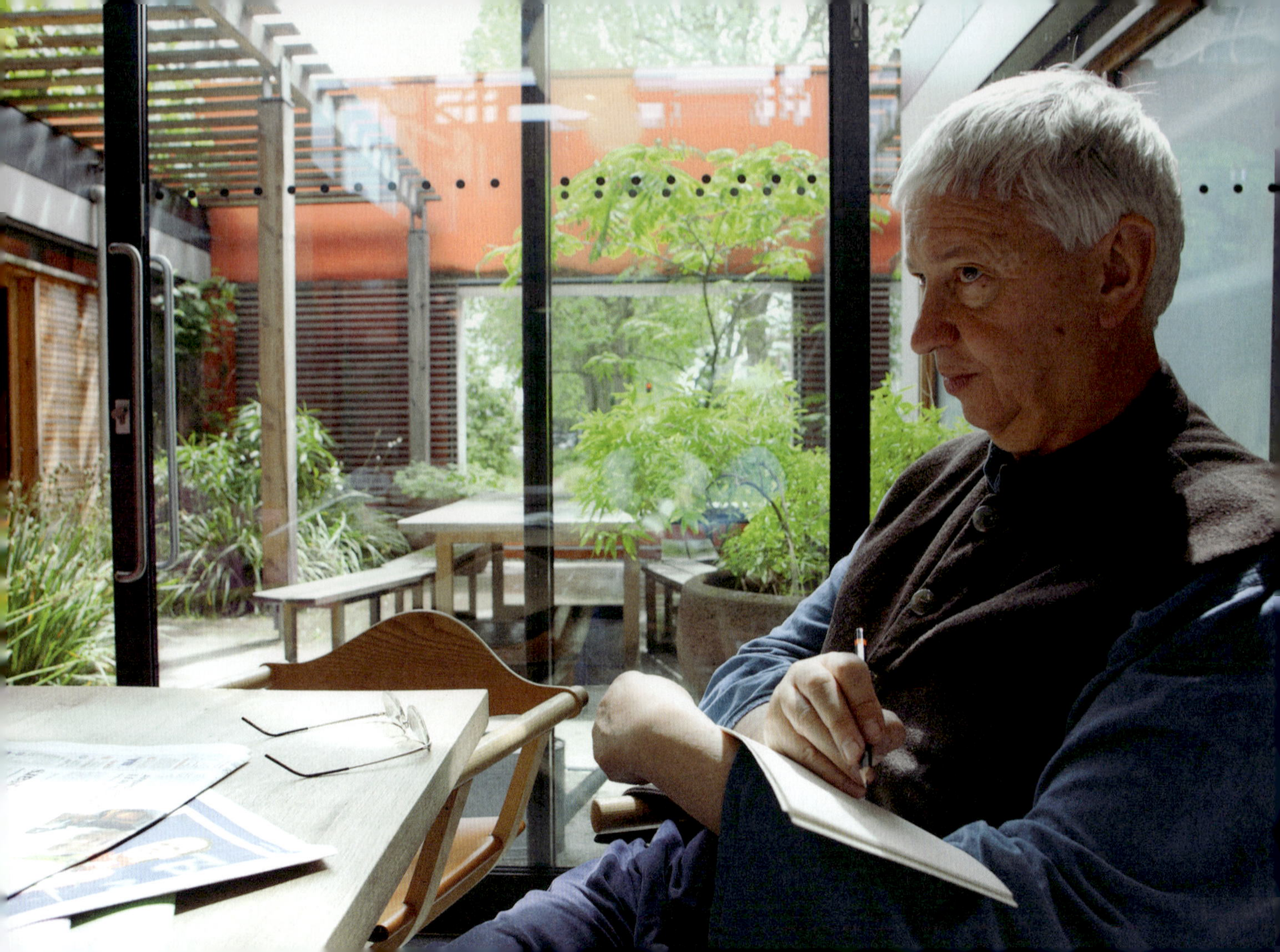

*Thursday 28 June*

I join the Oesophagus Cancer Group, but am asked not to draw during this first session. They are preoccupied above all with 'dumping', a kind of insulin-related gastric attack, especially terrible after the operation, and always unpredictable. The group is extremely varied in age, gender and ethnicity. All complain of the awful sense, having returned home from cancer surgery, of abandonment. There are no follow-up calls – a complete cut-off: 'It took me three weeks to recover a sense of worth.' I ask, 'Would it have helped if you'd been introduced to Maggie's before the surgery?' A resounding yes from all. Later, I sit and draw at the table, observing M at work. She later explains that she is conscious of her body language. Squatting on her heels beside a patient's chair might establish informality; kneeling shows concern and sympathy; when she stands, it is to show opposition to some form of unacceptable behaviour.

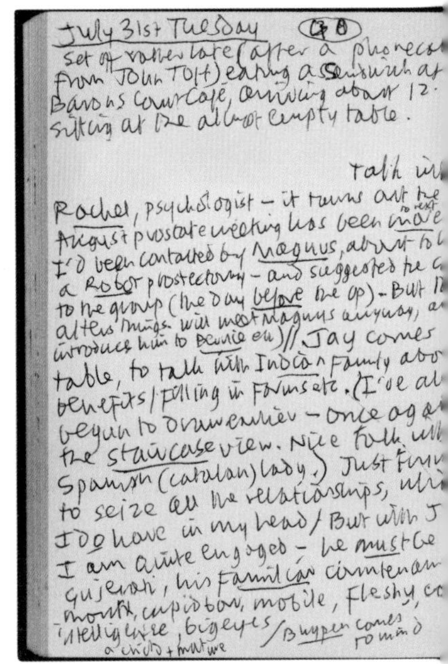

## JULY 2012

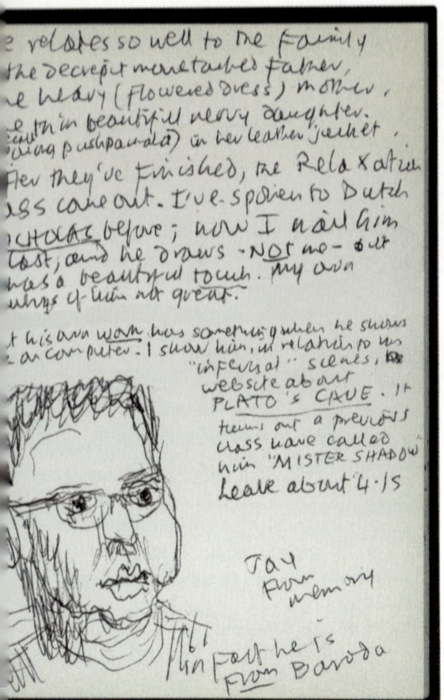


*Monday 2 July*
I wake feeling run down, with my left arm oddly aching. I have arranged to meet Jay at 11 am, and set off anyway. But his client never comes, and I hang about. Later I'm feeling exhausted so I shoot off.

*Tuesday 3 July*
After a bad night and severe cramp, I suddenly discover while taking my morning bath an enormous rash along my arm. It turns out to be shingles (*Herpes zoster*) and knocks me out for several days. But more significantly, even after what seems to be a recovery, I remain oddly depleted in energy, and vulnerable to other ailments. As Laura later emails me: 'Tim, you have to accept that shingles can be a six-month assault on the body.' The remaining months of my residency are indeed to be shadowed by this malaise. Judith and others wonder if my health has been undermined by my engagement with cancer, mortality, illness. (Shingles is usually stress-related.) Although I was enthusiastic about the Maggie's opportunity, and generally upbeat, had I been more inwardly affected than I'd realised?

*Thursday 26 July*
I enjoy my first day back, and the privilege of observing. But in the Oesophagus Group I'm careful not to draw those who seem most over-wrought or nervous.

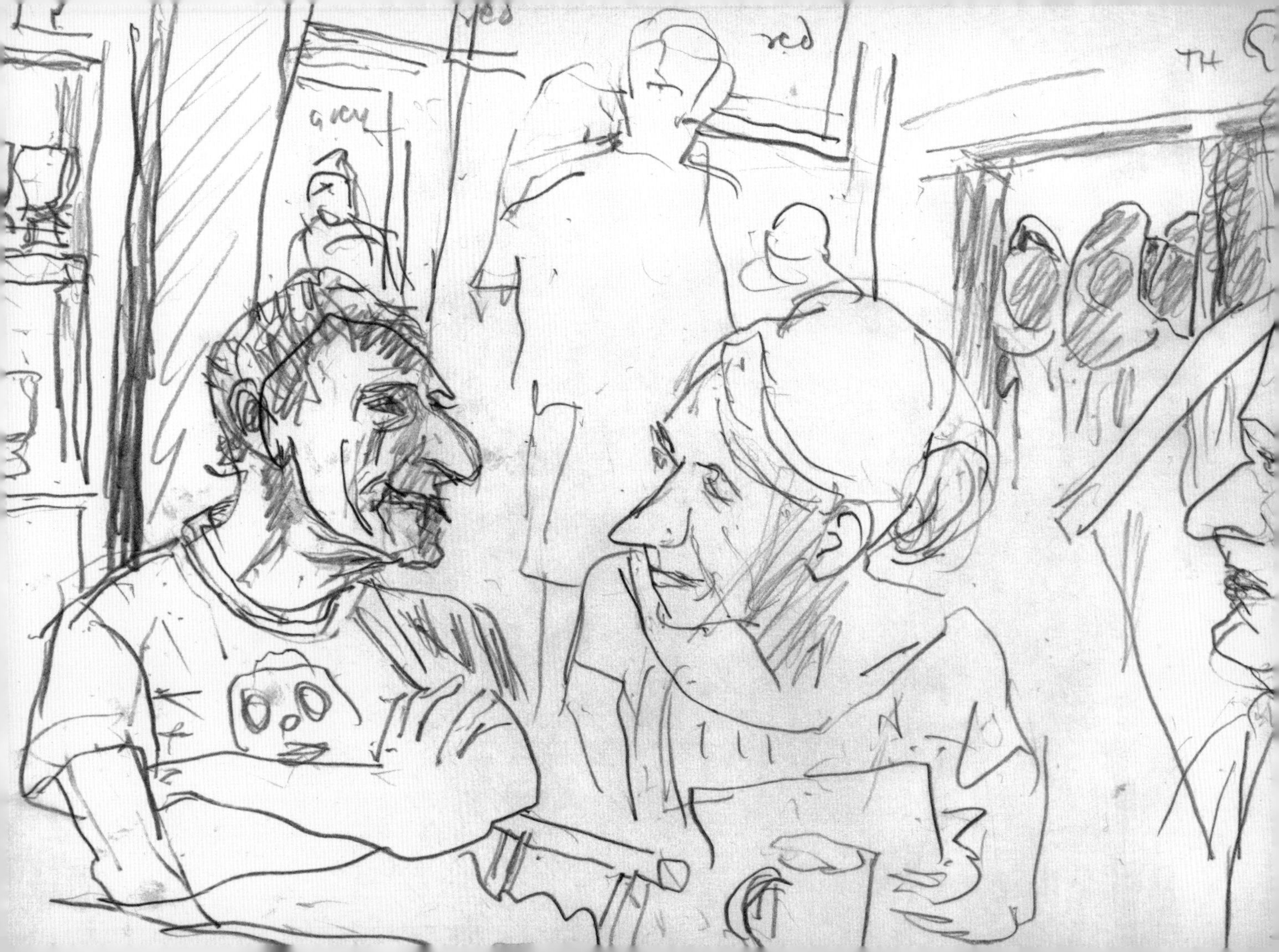
red
red
grey
TH

# AUGUST 2012

*Monday 6 August*

I've been contacted by my former studio comrade Magnus, who is about to have the new robot prostectomy. He has a black-humour blog, *The Cancer Times*. I introduce him to the Prostate Group, and draw him as he talks to Elaine. We eat together – my treat – a good meeting. On return, I get out pastels to make a colour study of the relationship between the stairs and the table (p. 76). I have delivered a folder of drawings for *Maggie's Matters*, the house magazine, and pencilled in a date for a presentation of my residency work, to be held in October at the National Portrait Gallery.

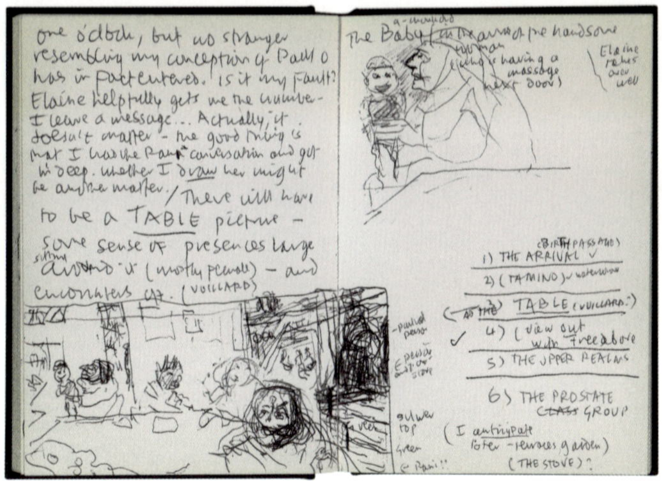

There will have to be a TABLE picture –
1) THE ARRIVAL ✓
TABLE (VUILLARD)
5) THE UPPER REALMS
6) THE PROSTATE GROUP
(THE STOVE)?


Magnus with Elaine

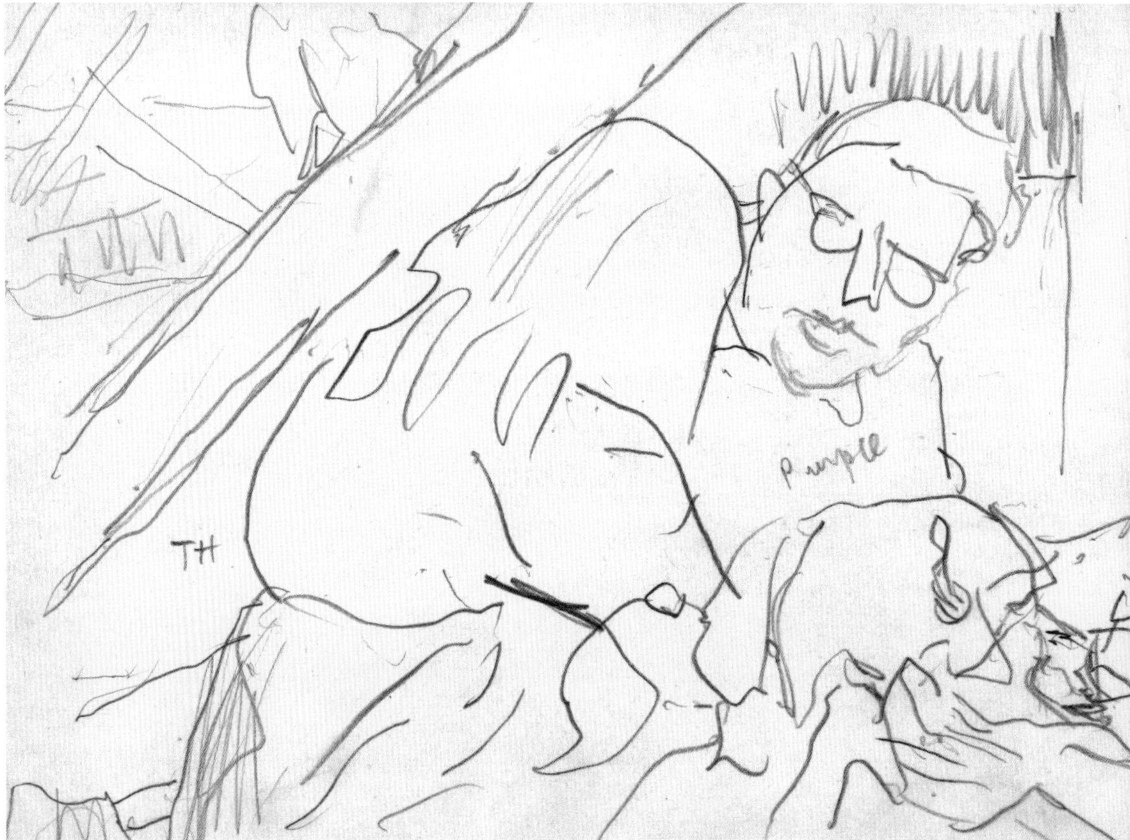
purple
TH

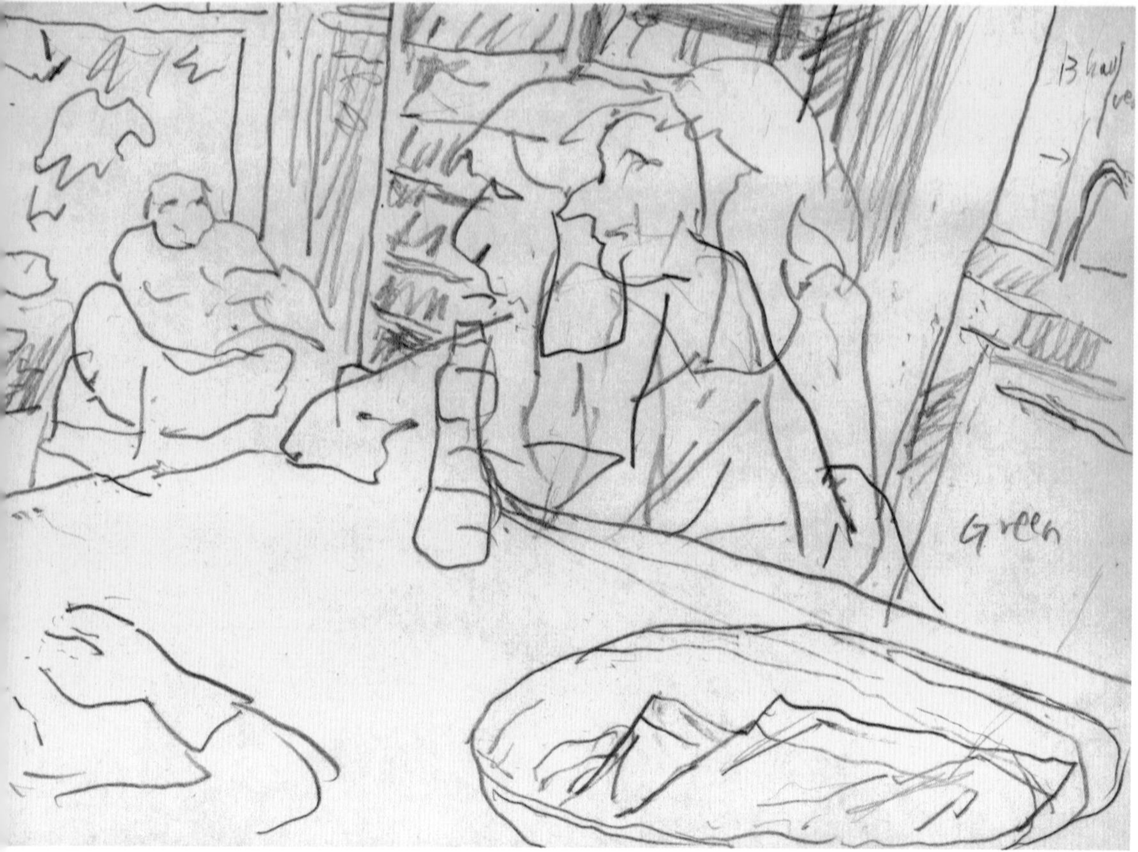


*Jay at the Table*

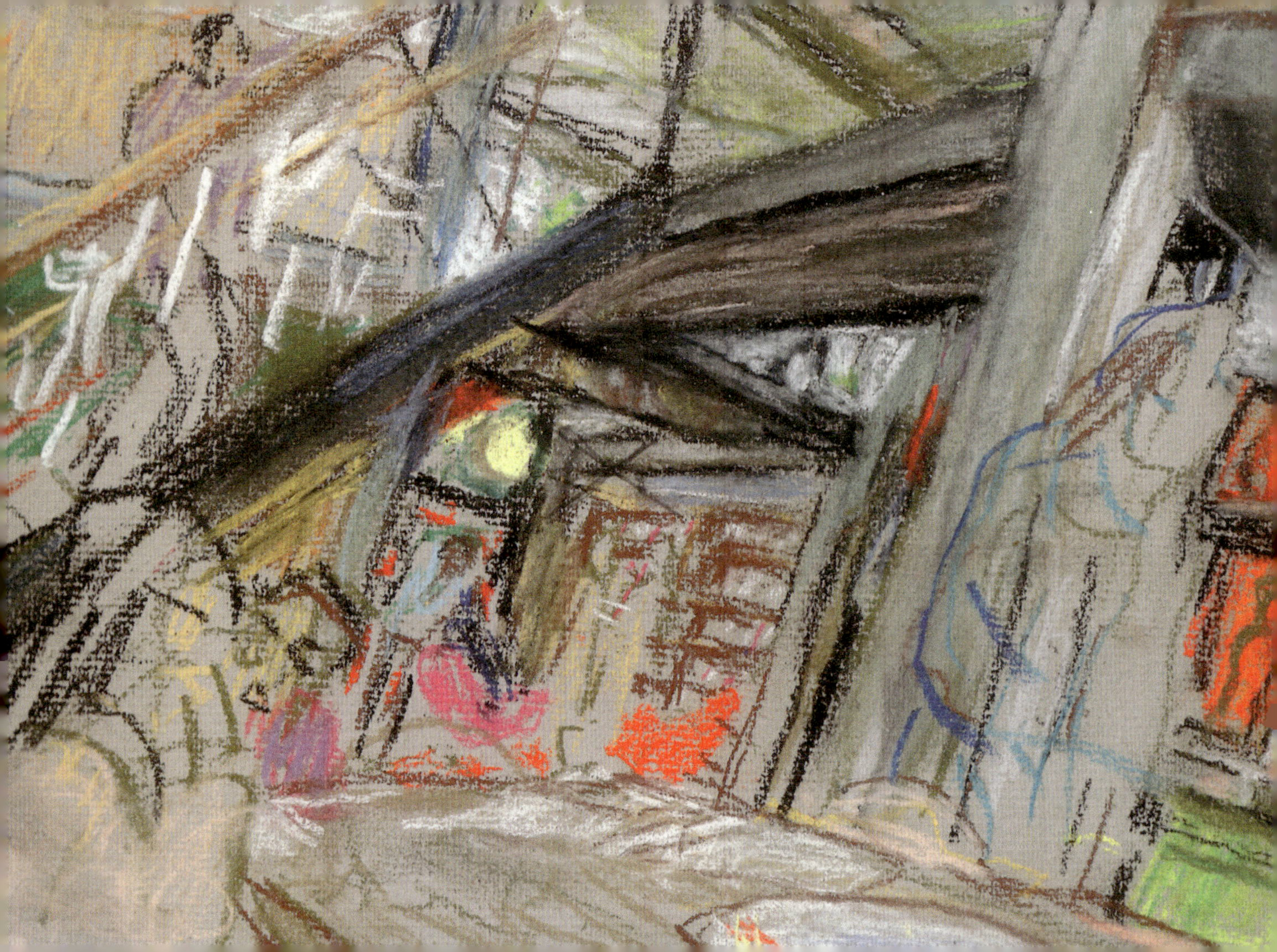

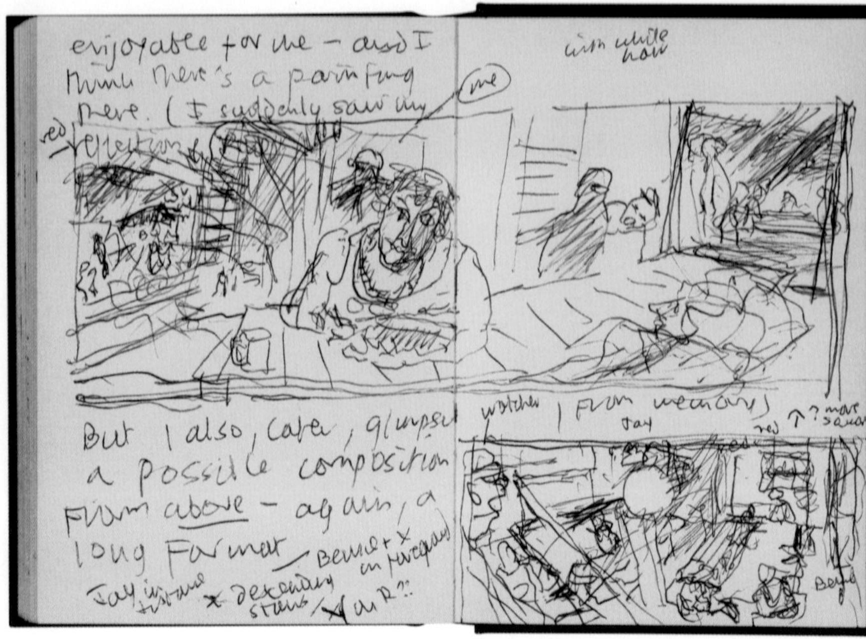
enjoyable for me – and I
think there's a painting
there. (I suddenly saw my
reflection
But I also, later, glimpse
a possible composition
from above – again, a
long format

*Tuesday 21 August*
After what is presumably another shingles aftermath – a horrible 'flu-like hiatus – I meet E and enjoy a good 90 minutes of mutual drawing in the garden. At one point I suddenly see my own reflection in the window – with white hair – over her shoulder, confirming there is a painting there.

LEFT *Jay, Stairs, Table*

OVERLEAF *E Drawing Me in the Courtyard*

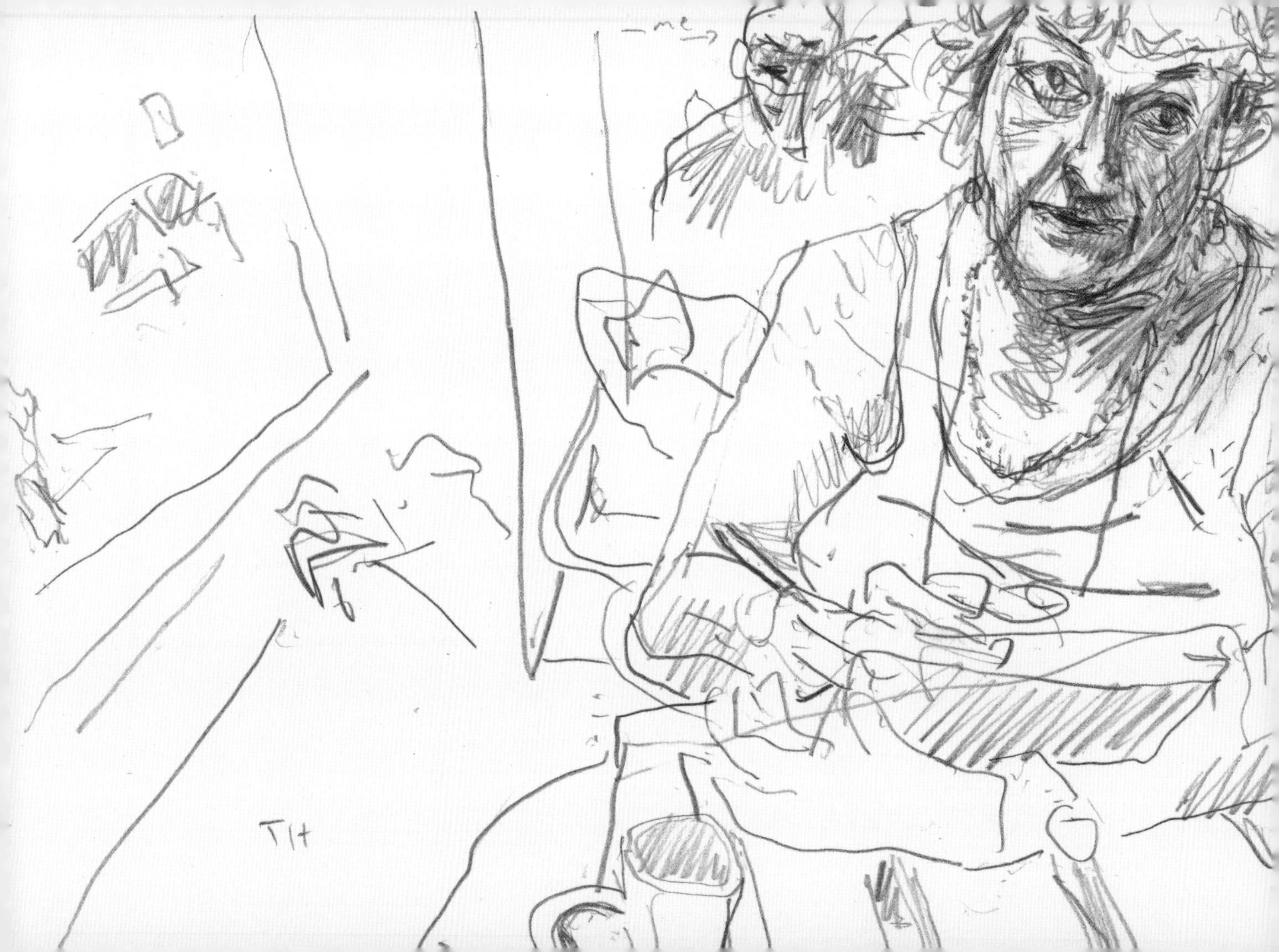
me

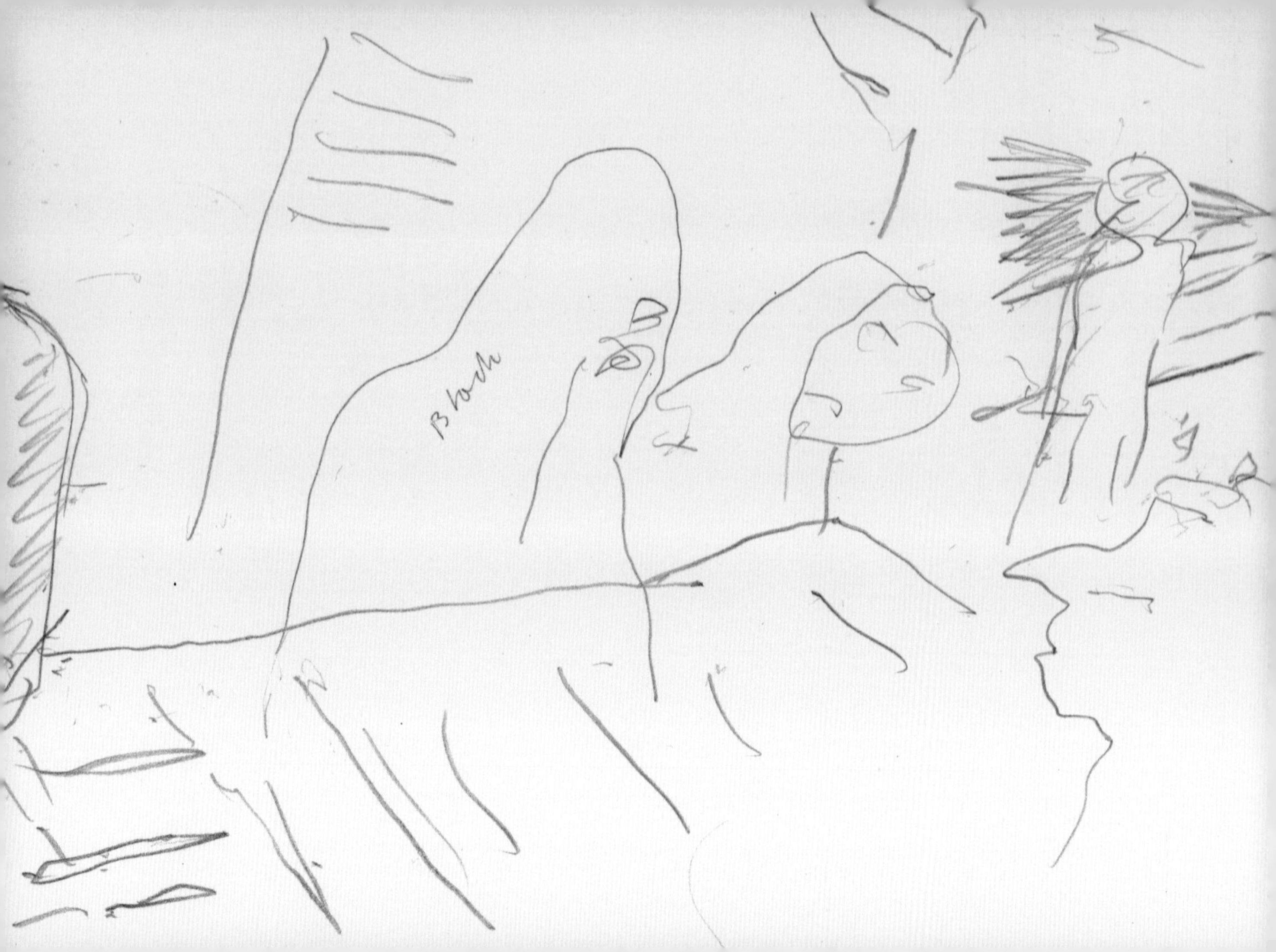
Bloch

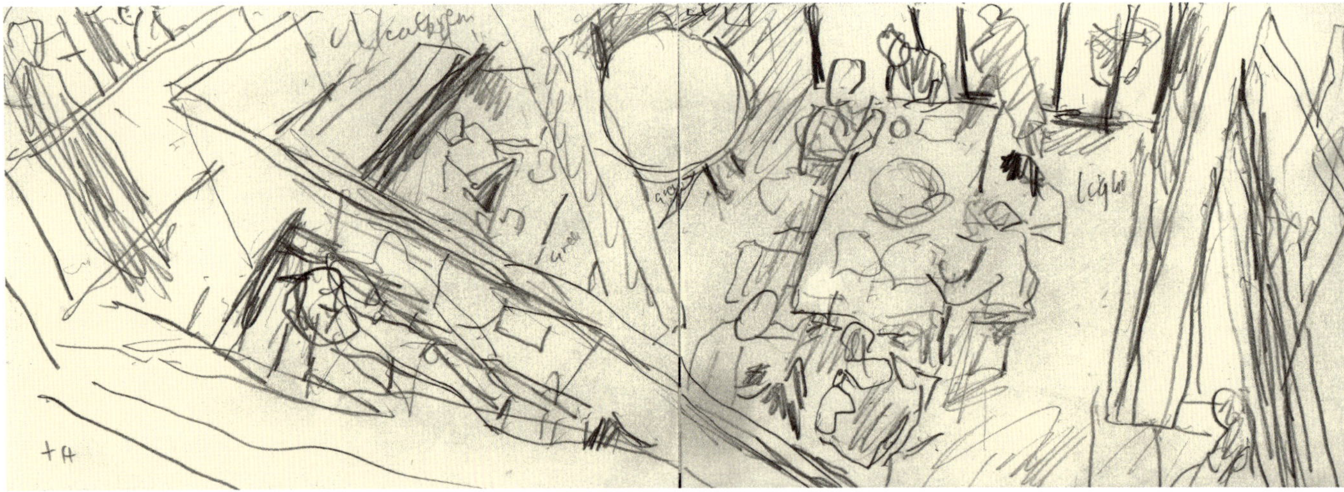

*Maggie's from Above I*

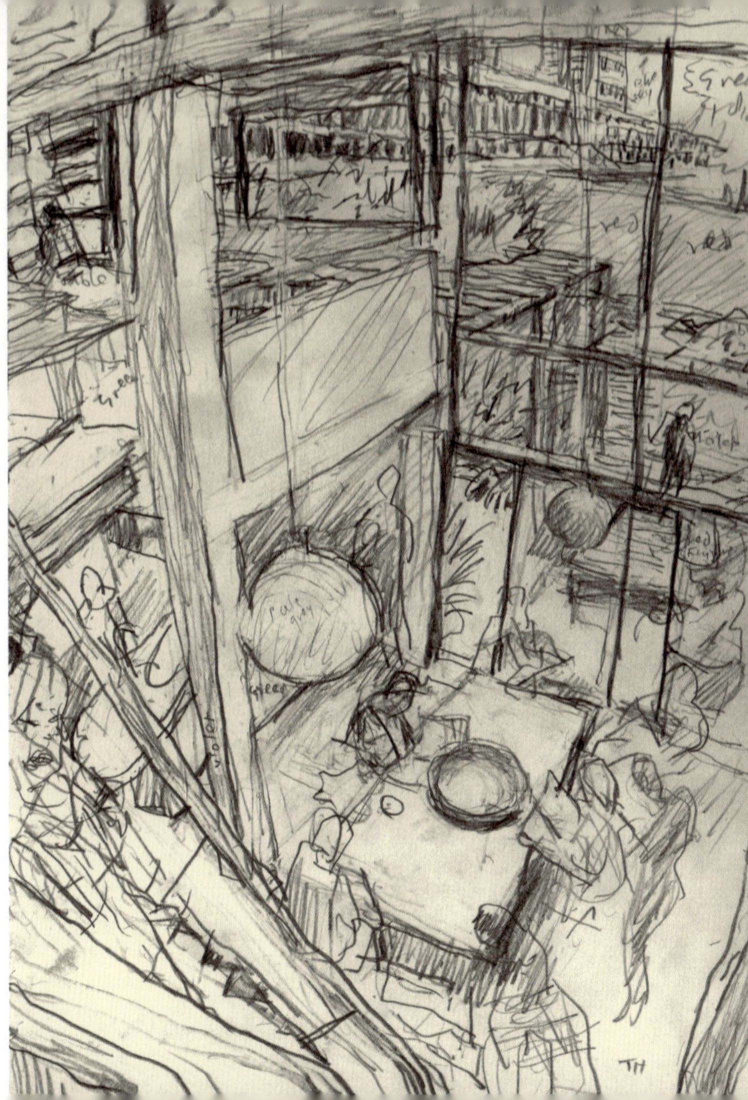


*Maggie's from Above II*

*Tuesday 28 August*
Upstairs, I take up my position, looking down onto the table, but this time within a vertical A4 format. Quite a tight, 'straight' drawing ensues (p. 81), of some intensity. I go down and talk with Nigel, and continue drawing when a staff-member comes to talk with him. I do feel sympathy – another operation for him tomorrow, he's had two and a half weeks in hospital, and lost a lot of blood. (Later, Elaine talks to me about shingles, and Mary advises acupuncture for exhaustion. As they point out, people *do* recover!)

## SEPTEMBER 2012

*Monday 3 September*
I meet up again with my friend Magnus, now post-op. He looks OK, although there are still massive complications for him. But when the Prostate Group assembles, the new psychologist informs me that, in her 'clinical judgement', I should not be present for the second part of the session, since 'palliative care' is such a loaded issue. Earlier, I'd drawn a good profile of piratical Chris.

*Tuesday 11 September*
I've been drawing E again in the garden space – a useful study through the window – and I have some sense that I now have enough information to make a possible portrait. I'm given excellent news about Rani – her brain tumour was not malignant, and she is still attending the Women's Group.

*Nigel*

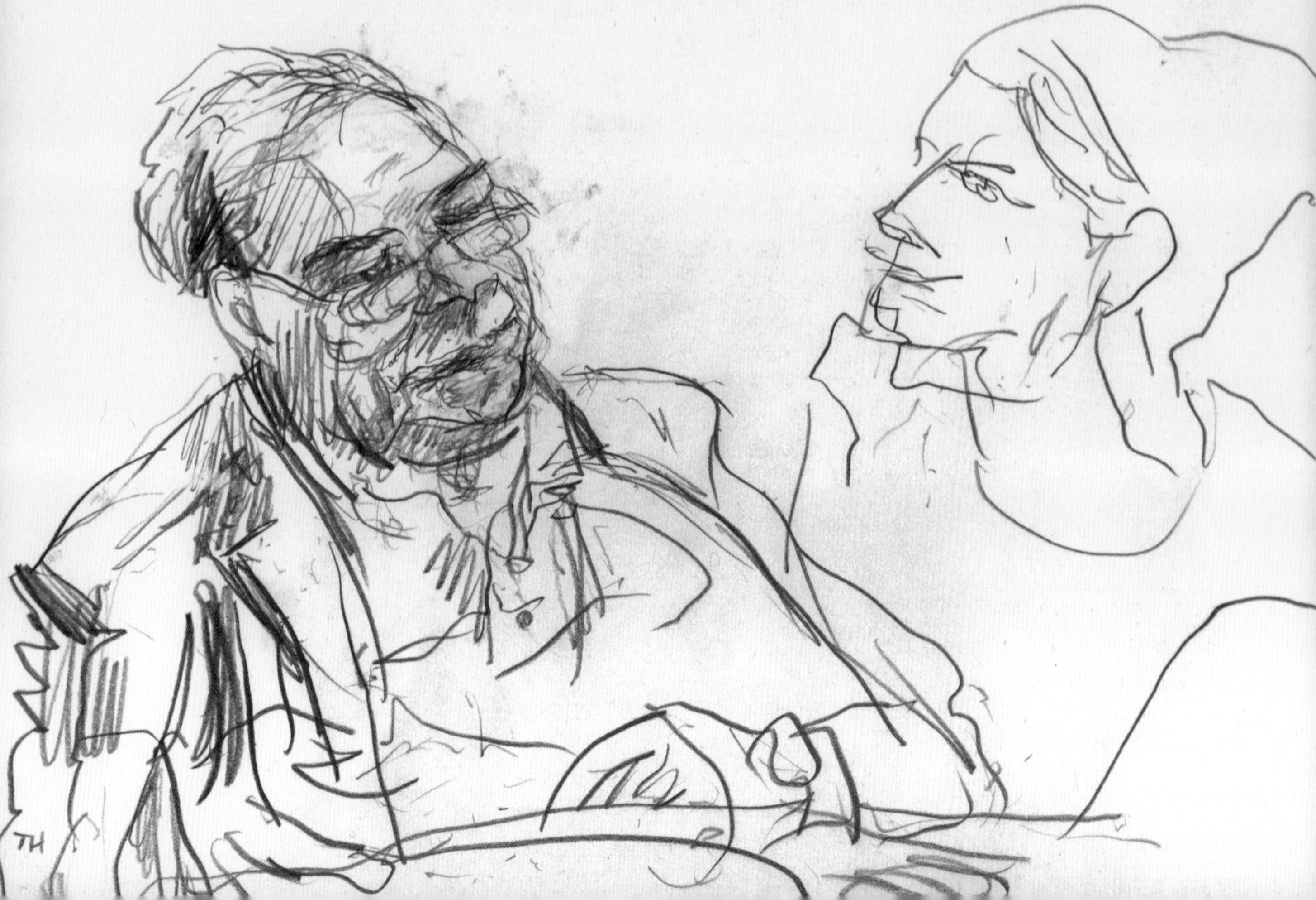
TH

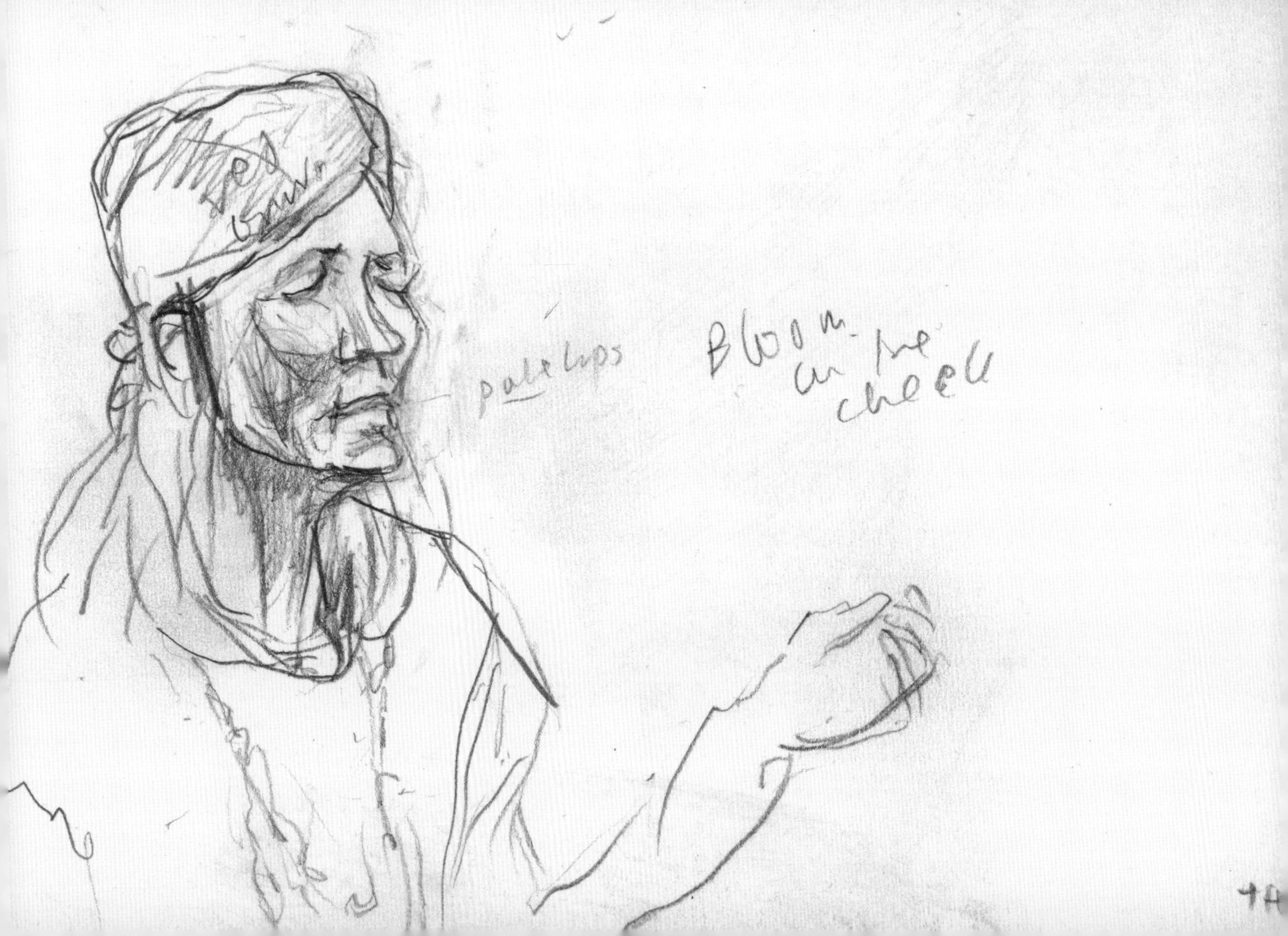
red brown
pale lips
Bloom on the cheek
4A

## OCTOBER 2012

*Tuesday 9 October*
I am trying to draw individuals, not very successfully. I draw the old Glaswegian who plays the piano at the hospital, doing his crossword at the table. Y says my drawing of her is not 'witchy' enough. Next day, Marie comes to the studio, to view the work so far, and I'm reassured by her quite enthusiastic response.

*Thursday 18 October*
I'm working better, drawing Nigel. Also reflections on glass, sudden cutaways, fragmented glimpses of sky. And this does help when I'm working at home on the paintings.

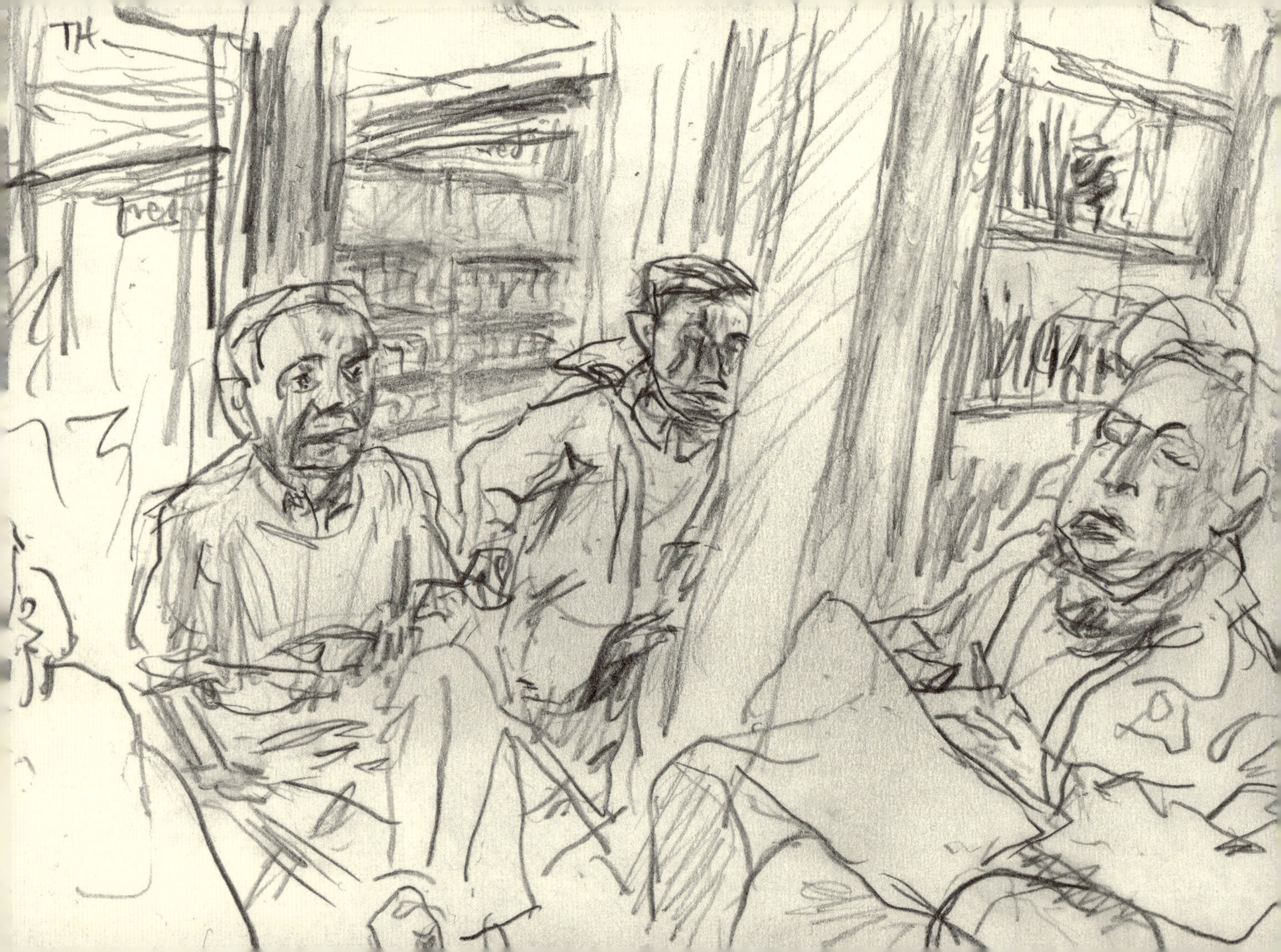
TH

*Monday 22 October*
I drew with Y again, less spooked; her own drawing, as always, is of quite high quality. My presentation of the residency takes place the following day, at the NPG. When I tell Sandy Moffat about the line-up of the committee I'm meeting there – including Sandy Nairne, Richard Calvocoressi, Charles Jencks, MaryAnne Stevens, Richard Cork, Laura Lee and several others – he emails back: 'My God! You're being hauled before the Spanish Inquisition.'

*Tuesday 23 October*
I have half an hour for my presentation. I take about 35 drawings, selected to give them the narrative of the residency so far. It goes fine, though I'm very knocked out by it.

## NOVEMBER 2012

*Monday 5 November*
I have a good drawing session at the Prostate Group, with a very lively, no-holds-barred discussion. I felt half-guilty at not joining the three men round the table afterwards – I like them – but I'm teaching a night drawing class at 6.30 pm.

*Tuesday 13 November*
I'm starting to stand back, to wind down. Drew E, perhaps for the last time.

*The Prostate Group VII*

*Thursday 29 November*

Alexey, a Red Cross volunteer, has agreed with Ernest, an 85-year-old, that I can draw while he is being massaged. Unfortunately I have only a very short session – but I enjoy it. As Elaine explains, most massage is for women, in crisis, and they refuse to be drawn. Then I return to paint in the studio.

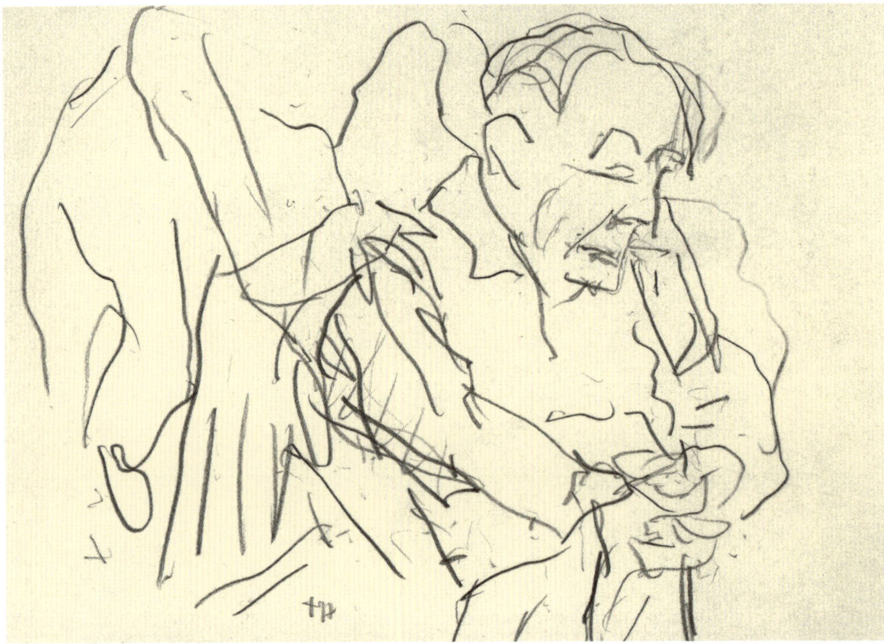

*Ernest Being Massaged I, II*

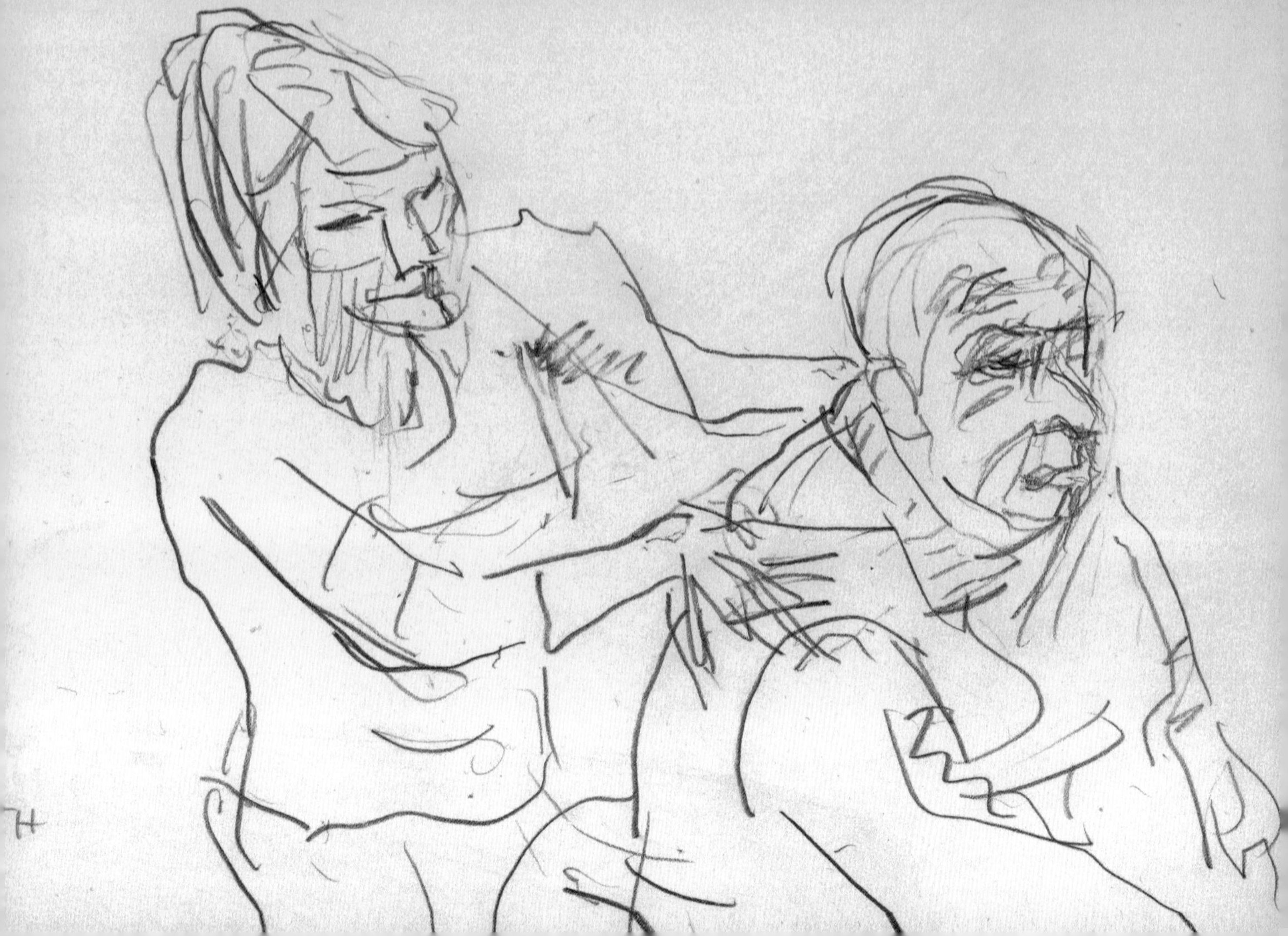

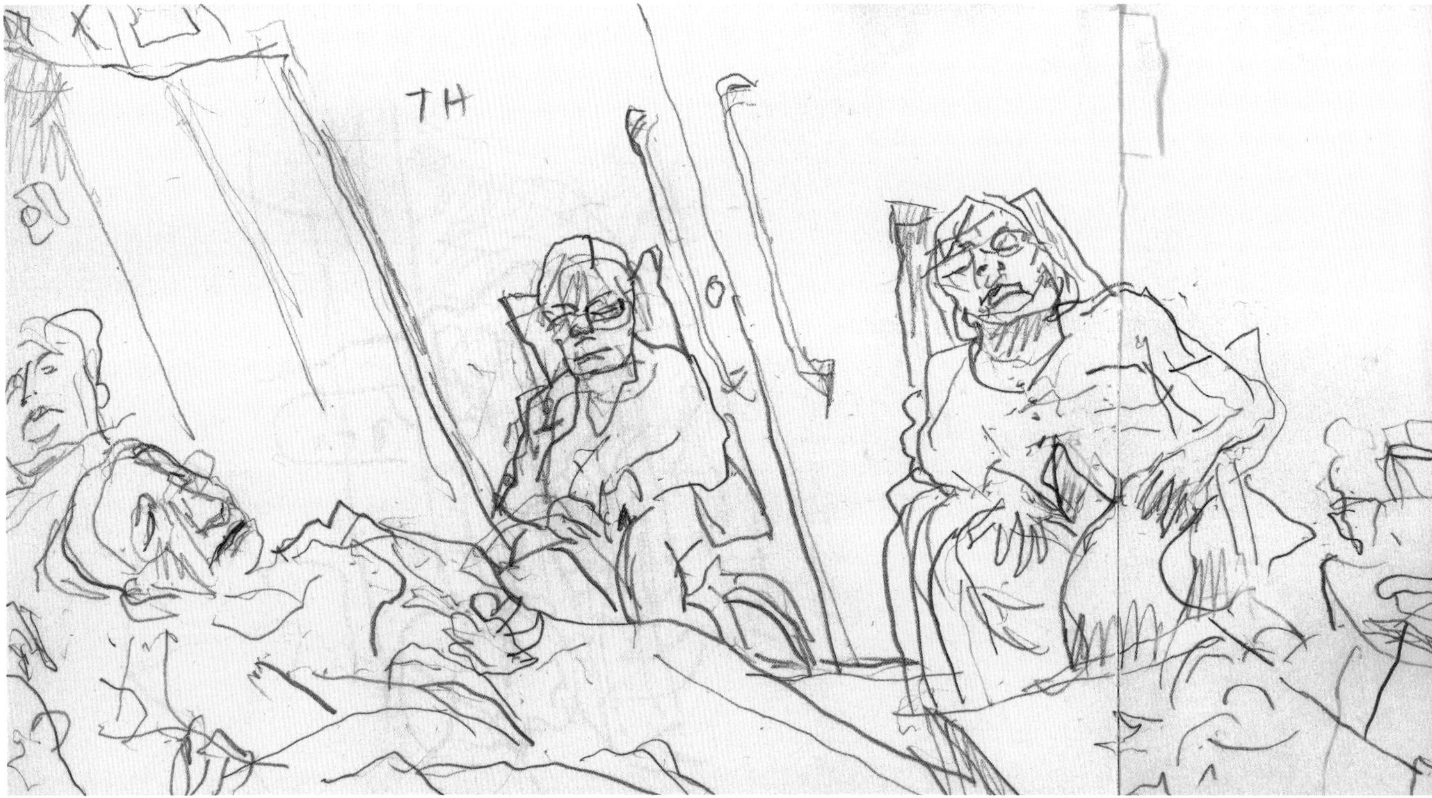


*Kirkcaldy Relaxation*

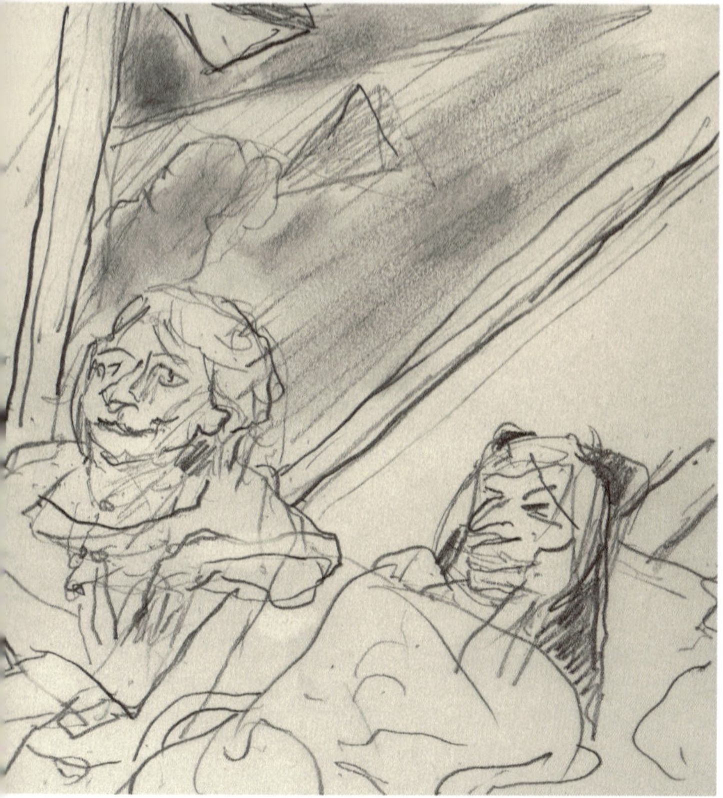

## DECEMBER 2012

*Tuesday 4 December*
With Sandy again, I travel by train to Kirkcaldy in Fife, and take a taxi up to the huge hospital. In front of it stands a little black painted pavilion, which looks at first not at all prepossessing, but this turns out to be Zaha Hadid's Maggie's Centre. (Later we'll hear of users calling it 'The Coffin', or 'The Ship of Death' or the 'Stealth Bomber'.) Yet the moment we enter, it is white and luminous with curves everywhere, a conscious shape-making in contrast to the *forced* acute angles of the exterior. As with most of the Maggie's Centres, Kirkcaldy is something of a woman's realm (Sandy: 'It's good to see women in charge for a change'). I keep on drawing at the table throughout, also attending a relaxation class, whose fantasy scenario is somehow recited more convincingly here than in London.

*Wednesday 5 December*
I travel to Dundee on my second visit. I want to focus this time on Gehry's interior, especially on the wooden flaps that come down from on high like tender, protective wings.

I station myself standing in the main room, drawing the whole, surprisingly large space on three A5 sheets. But the scale seems too miniaturised and I switch to A4. After lunch I draw a yoga class in a side room with a beautiful, curved wooden ceiling, and behind, a fine panoramic etching several feet long by the young Grayson Perry. Then I go back to my big drawing of the interior, as the room fills with mostly elderly people, all interacting enjoyably. Unknown to me, Sandy has been drawing me drawing.

*Thursday 20 December*
Having worked well at home on paintings, I arrive at about lunchtime for this second Maggie's Christmas party, and draw enjoyably from above, with the room already filling up. I am shocked to see Nigel enter, shuffling with a stick, very much worse. After an hour, I join the mêlée. It seems Nigel now has lung cancer; he was going to be operated on today, but it has been cancelled. I draw on, keeping him in sight…

My year with Maggie's has been among the most privileged experiences of my art-life, and I want to dedicate these drawings to the extraordinarily courageous individuals I encountered – both staff and 'users'.

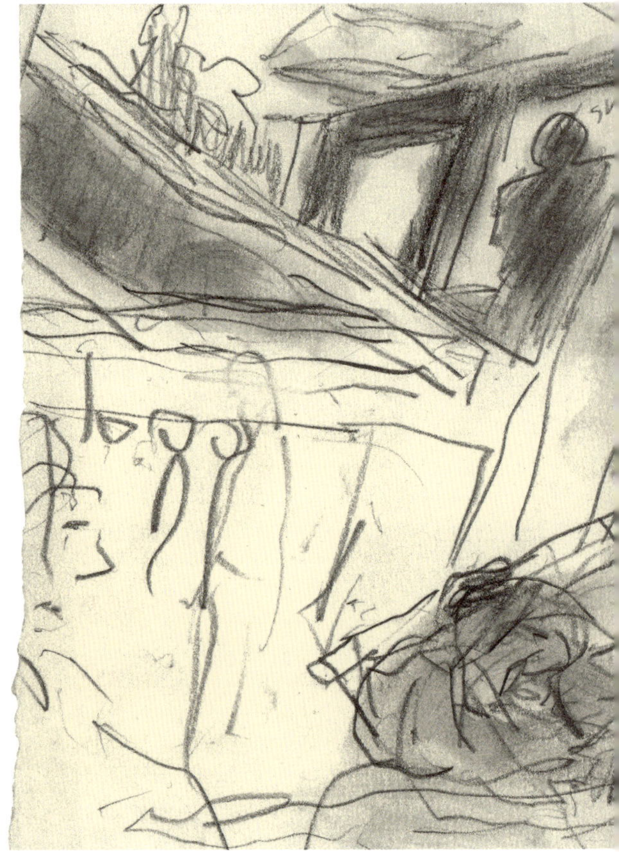

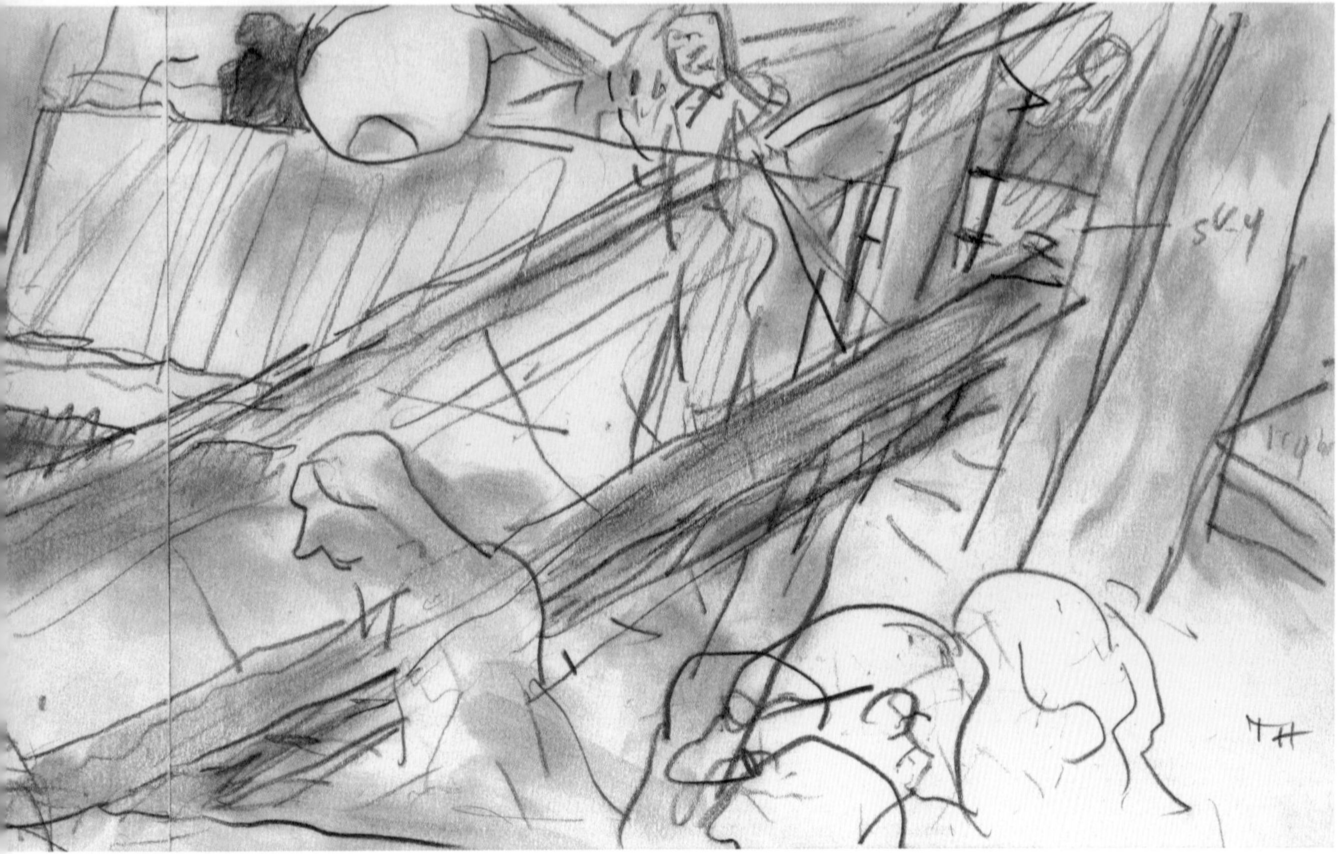


*Glimpses*

OVERLEAF *Interior of Gehry's Dundee*

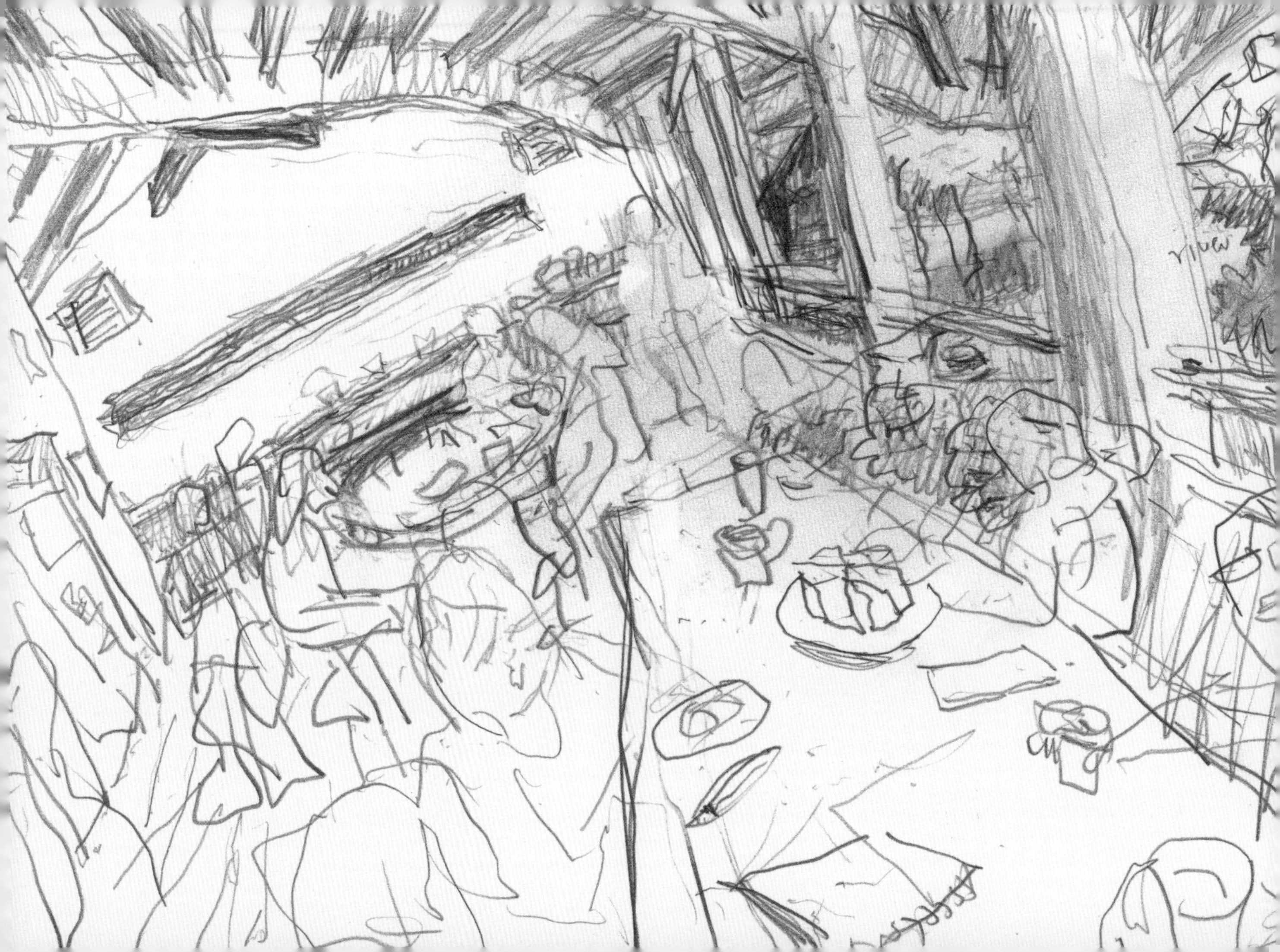
river

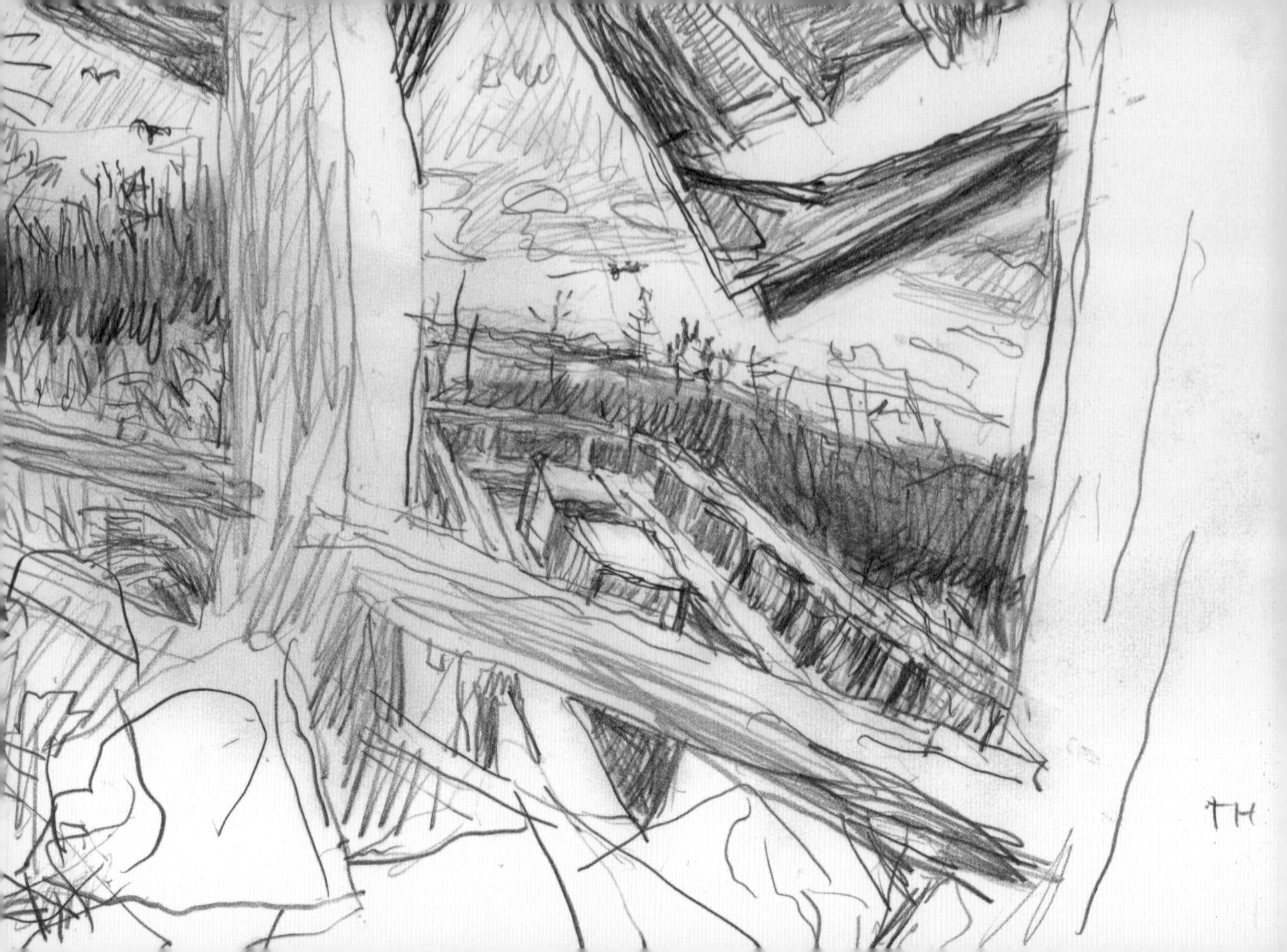
TH

This publication has been generously funded for Maggie's by the Cocheme Trust

ILLUSTRATIONS

Front cover: detail of *The Prostate Group III* (pages 30–31)

Back cover, pages 2, 68–69: the artist at the Maggie's Centre, Charing Cross Hospital, 21 June 2012. Photography by Philipp Ebeling

Page 4: detail of *Maggie's from Above II* (page 81)

*Royal Academy Publications*
Beatrice Gullström
Alison Hissey
Carola Krueger
Simon Murphy
Peter Sawbridge
Nick Tite

Design: Maggi Smith
Photography of artworks: DawkinsColour, London; John Bodkin
Colour origination: DawkinsColour, London

Printed by Conti Tipocolor, Florence, Italy



British Library Cataloguing-in-Publication Data
A catalogue record for this book is available from the British Library
ISBN 978-1-907533-96-9

Distributed outside the United States and Canada
by Thames & Hudson Ltd, London